THE ENTHUSIASM–
LAFFTER CONNECTION

THE ENTHUSIASM-LAFFTER CONNECTION

A Guide for Gaining Positive Life Skills

Bob "Hubba Jubba" Moss

Motivation Lecturer, Coach, and Mentor

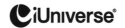

THE ENTHUSIASM–LAFFTER CONNECTION
A Guide for Gaining Positive Life Skills

iUniverse books may be ordered through booksellers or by contacting:

iUniverse
1663 Liberty Drive
Bloomington, IN 47403
www.iuniverse.com
1-800-Authors (1-800-288-4677)

*Because of the dynamic nature of the Internet, any web addresses or
links contained in this book may have changed since publication and
may no longer be valid. The views expressed in this work are solely those
of the author and do not necessarily reflect the views of the publisher,
and the publisher hereby disclaims any responsibility for them.*

*Any people depicted in stock imagery provided by Thinkstock are models,
and such images are being used for illustrative purposes only.
Certain stock imagery © Thinkstock.*

ISBN: 978-1-4917-6528-9 (sc)
ISBN: 978-1-4917-6529-6 (e)

Library of Congress Control Number: 2015905579

Print information available on the last page.

iUniverse rev. date: 06/30/2015

The enthusiasm–laffter connection has been very, very good to me!
(Bob Hubba Jubba Moss)

This book is first dedicated to my immediate family, including my parents, the late LaVerne and Robert Clinton Moss Sr.; my wife, Edna Jean; my brother, Oliver, and his family; my children, Anita Young (and her husband, Grayelin) and Parry; and my grandchildren, Aladrianne and Junior. Also, I dedicate this work to other relatives, colleagues, and students who have enjoyed and respected my passion for sharing enthusiasm–laffter lessons!

Table of Contents

About the Author

Bob "Hubba Jubba" Moss

Motivation Lecturer, Coach and Mentor,

Volunteer Motivation Coach University of Arkansas Pine Bluff (2006- Present)

Formerly:
Adjunct Faculty, University of Arkansas Pine Bluff (2008-2010); Teacher, Coach & Counselor, San Diego Unified School District (1965- 1971 and 1995- 2001 [Retired 2000]); Physical Education Department, Faculty Emeritus, University of California San Diego (UCSD); (1971-92); US Marine Corps (1961-65).

Bob Moss was born, raised and educated in San Diego, California. In 2006 he moved to White Hall, Arkansas 34 miles south of Little Rock, and a mile north of Pine Bluff. Over the past 45 years, he has developed a unique passion establishing joyous and enthusiastic attitudes for person of all ages.

Moss holds degrees and/or credentials from San Diego State University (BA & MA) and Cal Western University (teaching credentials). He has given decades of leadership services to the local, state, regional and national affairs of professional organization, in the areas of physical education and counselor education. His professional leadership efforts have included conference presentation, in-service workshops and keynote addresses. He has received many peer awards for his dedicated professional involvements. He is also praised for his role as a drum major for urging greater professional involvement by diverse educators.

Referred to by friends, students and colleagues as "Hubba Jubba" Moss is highly regarded for his presentations promoting enthusiasm and joy for others. While teaching at UCSD, Moss utilized his classroom as a laboratory for developing visualization techniques allowing students to experience accelerated learning of motor skills and attitudes. Combining his talent as a self-styled enthusiastic sports official with a gamut of visualization techniques, he assisted students to become high level referees and umpires in a very short period of time.

By chance in the late 1970's, Moss stumbled across the relationship between his enthusiastic mannerism and "Gelotology" (the study of laffter). Hence the "laffter/enthusiasm" concept was born. Moreover, Bob has pioneered the role of "sports motivation coach" since 1972, and has served as a consultant at all levels of sports play, across America and on several West Indies Islands. He also often times speaks on the topic: "Transcending Multicultural Barriers."

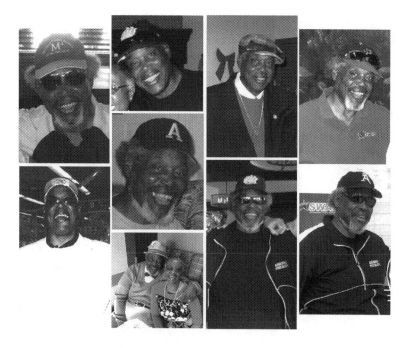

Foreword

By: Dr. Jack Douglass
Retired, University of California San Diego, Vice Chancellor,
Researcher and Faculty Member

I am proud and happy to contribute a few thoughts regarding the written works of my colleague and good friend Bob "Hubba Jubba" Moss. On so many occasions, I have described Bob as an "experience getting ready to happen." In the spring of 1971, while serving as a vice chancellor at UCSD, I informed Bob of an open faculty position in our physical education department. Moss was a high school teacher, coach, and counselor at the time of his interview, and he was hired from a slate of highly qualified candidates. He immediately began establishing himself as one of the most dynamic and student-friendly teachers on campus. During my tenure at UCSD, I frequently shared the fact Bob Moss was one of the most creative and student-friendly faculty members on campus!

In the spring of 1992, Bob Moss retired from UCSD with faculty emeritus honors and continued teaching at the local high school and elementary school levels for another ten years. After retiring once again, he continued his classroom presence as the "Hubba Jubba Subba" until he and his bride of fifty-three years (Edna) relocated to White Hall, Arkansas, in 2006. The validity of Hubba Jubba's successful ventures are made obvious by the quality and quantity of his lectures and workshop presentations to state and national professional organizations, K–12 schools, institutions of higher education, professional and intercollegiate athletic teams, and community groups.

So what's so special about Hubba Jubba's creative and friendly ventures? First of all, during his second year at UCSD, he added the concept of mental imagery to his tennis class syllabus, creating a scientific reach allowing students to gain personal experiences with academic theory seldom available in their scientific and mathematics classrooms. Thanks to their mental imagery (or "pretend practice") lessons, most students were awed by the accelerated improvement of their tennis skills. Moss immediately expanded the concept to his softball classes and sport officiating course, his work with student athletes, and then an "accelerated improvement of motor skills" course, funded by a UC Regents instruction improvement grant.

Secondly, the combination of Bob's spirited attitude, rotund body mass, and jovial personality enables him to immediately connect with others. Late in his second teaching year at UCSD, he began to realize his natural enthusiasm had been at the root of his ability to effectively communicate with his students.

Just a few years later, Moss stumbled across the subject of gelotology (the study of laffter). When combined with enthusiasm instruction, this served as a unique motivational teaching approach; thus the enthusiasm–laffter connection began.

It has been a valued professional and personal treat to observe the growth and progressive development of Bob's motivational talents from the UCSD tennis courts to Arkansas, where he now resides. Over the years, Moss has eagerly served as a professional and community leader, always ready to share his creative motivational presentations with others; in fact, the world. My most memorable times with Bob occurred over four summers during which I included him on my touring team of physical educators providing tennis lessons for youths and their teachers on the West Indies islands of Saint Thomas, Saint Croix, Saint Lucia, and Barbados. In addition to his tennis clinic duties, Bob volunteered numerous motivation presentations to the staff and guests at our host hotels, to national sport teams, to summer youth camps, and to health groups. It was a joy watching him immediately gain heartwarming respect from the island people as they responded to his extreme gestures of laffter and enthusiasm. Moreover, two of our summers in Barbados found Bob receiving standing ovations after singing his Louie Armstrong rendition (raspy voice and all) of "Hello Dolly" during the island's traditional pre-carnival Crop Over calypso concerts.

I close by informing readers that the concepts, ideas, and images in this book were mainly conceived through Bob's "the classroom is my laboratory" approach for enhancing the quality of his teaching and mentoring endeavors. His outside-the-box focus is demonstrated in the discussion of such topics as "enthusiasm is a learnable skill," "anatomy of hearty laffter," "no smiles or grins," "handmade remember 2B positive mementos," "pretend practice activities," "mirror box drills," and "transcending multicultural barriers."

Preface

The Enthusiasm–Laffter Connection spotlights decades of joy I have experienced from teaching, promoting, and mentoring enthusiasm as a valuable life skill. It is amazing to find that a characteristic as important as human enthusiasm is rarely found in the curricula of schools, employee training programs, professional workshops, and management seminars. In the past, writers frequently spoke on the values of an enthusiastic personality but failed to explain how it can be acquired and maintained. Currently, more and more media references appear on the healthy benefits of laffter. Today folks everywhere are burdened by any variety of stressful situations, including concerns for financial obligations, family strife, and job security. More than ever before, we are in dire need of ways to deal with the adversities and frustrations in our lives. So fret no more, readers; here comes *The Enthusiasm–Laffter Connection* to save the day!

The topics appearing in this book evolved from a 50 year career teaching biology, coaching sport teams, designing tennis visualization drills, and promoting hearty laffter as the best enthusiasm. The first sign of my eventual ties with enthusiasm was indicated when my parents nicknamed me Buzzy because I was always as "busy as a buzzing bee." Through my K–12 and college education, I continued buzzing along as an athlete and student held in high esteem by peers. Following graduation from San Diego State University (1961), I served four years in the US Marine Corps, where I played football for the San Diego Marine Corps Depot (MCRD) and applied my artistic abilities (I was an art minor in college) as a training aids illustrator and football team sign painter. A most interesting event in my US Marine career occurred when I was transferred overseas to the US Marine Corps detachment on Coronado Island, just a half mile from downtown San Diego.

After my years in the US Marine Corps, I became a high school teacher, coach, and counselor. My avid teaching personality was an immediate hit with the students I influenced. At the same time, I became involved as a football, basketball, and baseball and softball official, which led to three summers of Minor League Baseball umpiring in Montana, Idaho, Utah, and California. Through my referee and umpiring services, I became noted for my "more enthusiastic than others" approach to sports officiating. My body mechanics and verbal gestures were patterned in the style of the late Emmett Ashford, who was the first African American to umpire in Major League Baseball. Emmett became my close friend and mentor, and I was in awe with pride when a news article likened me to a giant economy-sized Emmett Ashford. While I failed to realize it at the time, my innovative flare for officiating would lead to the beginning of my academic involvement with efforts of enthusiasm instruction.

The summer of 1971 marked the end of my three-year dream to become a Major League umpire. Umpire development administrators felt my extreme gestures were no more than hotdogging or showboating and were not what they were looking for in a Major League prospect. (Anyone remember the old Charlie the Tuna commercials?) I was completely devastated by the news, and for the second time in my life I came face-to-face with the age old adage "Out of heartbreak and sorrow, seeds of something greater will come to pass." In late August 1971, I found out I had been hired as a physical education faculty member at the University of California San Diego (UCSD). To tell the truth, I felt a bit uneasy during my first fall quarter teaching beginning tennis and softball classes, mainly because of the highly intelligent background of UCSD students.

During the second term, I ran across two books that literally changed my life. I combined the knowledge gained from reading *Think and Grow Rich* (Napoleon Hill) and *Psycho-Cybernetics* (Maxwell Maltz) to develop a theoretical approach to tennis success. Through the design of teaching techniques emphasizing positive mental images and pretend practice drills, I enabled students to accelerate the learning of their skills beyond their wildest expectations.

During the 1972 spring term, due to a campus-wide budget cutback, our athletic department had to release funds back to the general campus budget, and my department administrators challenged me to prepare my officiating class students to officiate the bases, while one local umpire (rather than two) would be assigned to home plate duties. The college umpiring group refused to cooperate with the plan, so I resigned and pursued the challenge of training student officials to umpire the games played by their varsity baseball team. The students in my Psychology of Sports Officiating course used visualization (pretend practice) drills to empower themselves with accelerated officiating skills in just a few weeks' time. For eight baseball seasons, my student officials umpired all UCSD baseball games. We also umpired the varsity schedules played by the San Diego State University baseball team for two seasons (1974 and 1975). Never before and never again will student officials have the opportunity to enjoy such advanced officiating experiences!

Within a year, the officiating class became a smashing hit on campus, and many students enrolled just to sit in on the positive vibes the class provided, while never officiating a single athletic event. Student officials expanded their interests to other sports, such as volleyball, swimming, tennis, basketball, ice hockey, and soccer. Selected students assumed duties coordinating and administering umpire programs for local youth and adult leagues, as well as working local high school and community college sport contests. Over a twenty-year period, officiating class participants earned more than $3.5 million in officiating fees, and dozens of students financed their college education through yearlong officiating activities. During this time, umpire interns filled the void caused by large numbers of adult umpires employed as construction workers on the Trans-Alaska Pipeline project.

While the officiating course grew in popularity, I began to share news of the officiating program's success at meetings of professional organizations, as it was the most popular choice on the UCSD chancellor's speaking bureau. I was one of two faculty members selected to have their students visit with noted financial contributors at quarterly chancellor colloquium presentations. Early in the 1980s I stumbled across the thought that hearty laffter is the grandest gesture of enthusiasm. Since then I have progressively developed actions and attitudes encouraging others to gain and maintain high levels of enthusiasm and healthy laffter on a 24-7 basis. All images appearing on these pages were created as visual aids for classroom lectures, motivation presentations, and university/community services. Regardless of your age or station in life, *The Enthusiasm–Laffter Connection* is for you.

The intent of this book is to provide readers with ideas and uses for the enthusiasm–laffter connection. All thoughts and activities are focused on the concept that hearty laffter is the greatest gesture of human enthusiasm. A major purpose of these materials is to provide in-depth looks at how to understand, develop, and sustain the lasting talent of eternal enthusiasm. Enthusiasm becomes a learned characteristics once you become aware of how important it is, how to get it, and how to maintain it as a 24-7 lifestyle activity.

The healthy values of laffter are increasing their presence as popular topics in current magazine, newspaper, and journal articles. Special attention is given to the fact that healthy and healing conditions are initiated only through the use of hearty and robust laffs—no smiles or grins allowed. Also, the anatomy of hearty laffter (what it looks and sounds like) is discussed, and many ideas are shared on how to put more laffter into our daily life experiences.

Also included are concepts on environmental management (the images appearing in your hallways and on your bedroom walls and personal items). By using handmade memento items encouraging "remember 2B positive" habits, along with the use of mental imagery drills (also known as creative visualization or pretend practice drills), one is able to achieve accelerated mind-expanding physical skills and personal attitudes.

Read and then actualize the ideas shared in *The Enthusiasm–Laffter Connection*, and find yourself rapidly becoming more successful at all you do!

Acknowledgments

So many teaching colleagues have influenced the continued development of my creative speaking, teaching, and motivation skills. A list of these persons would fill many pages, and a short list of names would omit many I owe depths of gratitude to. I tip my hat to the K–12 through higher education educators and all others who have recognized and supported my unique techniques for sharing gestures of enthusiasm and hearty laffter. Thank you, thank you, thank you all very much!

And to the students who I have associated with over the past fifty years, I commend you for your eagerness to learn and use the creative actions I encouraged you to understand. Oftentimes, I felt I was learning as much from you as you were learning from me.

And lastly, I give a hearty thanks to those who tried to sabotage my progress on various occasions, based upon my (1) robust body girth, (2) actions and ideas they could not or did not want to understand, (3) zest for demonstrating healthy and hearty laffter, and (4) dedicated commitment to advance and promote multicultural awareness. This last group's closed-mindedness, ignorance, and status-quo-forever gestures energized my desire to research, develop, model, and teach positive life skill learning adventures! To these narrow-minded nincompoops, contact me if you can; I owe you a six-pack of your favorite beverage!

Chapter 1

Enthusiasm:
Catch It, Learn It, Share It

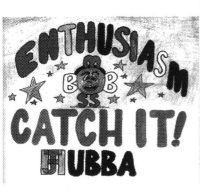
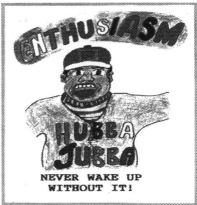

Enthusiasm is the greatest life skill we can develop. What our world needs now are organized efforts teaching concepts and techniques for gaining greater human enthusiasm. What does your enthusiasm look like?

People who have it can't really explain how they got it, do not know how to discuss it with others, and just hope they can keep it. Those lacking it marvel at those who have it and wish they could find some (maybe in their mailbox someday—ha!). The following pages are dedicated to the idea that enthusiasm can be taught.

It's hard to believe very few (if any) curricula are designed specifically to teach enthusiasm skills. Over the past four decades, I have pursued a deep passion for teaching and mentoring gestures of extreme enthusiasm. The organized instruction of enthusiasm is an idea whose time has come! An amazing quality of enthusiasm is its ability to cultivate positive feelings in those who have it. Be they at home, in the neighborhood, on the job, or at school, folks who exhibit major images of enthusiasm naturally draw others to them. What more people need to understand is that their enthusiasm, or lack of it, is constantly observed and evaluated by others. What does your enthusiasm look like? Do you even care? If you wanted to upgrade your personal enthusiasm, would you know how? Here are a few basic enthusiasm facts:

- Enthusiasm is a learnable skill.
- In the beginning, you must learn to "fake it to make it."
- Great leaders share their enthusiasm with others.
- Exhibited enthusiasm encourages enhanced excellence.
- Hearty laffter is the best tool to aid enthusiasm learning.

**ENTHUSIASM: NAME FOR GAME OF LIFE;
HEARTY LAFFS ARE THE BEST ENTHUSIASM
AT FIRST FAKE IT TO LEARN IT
STAY SURROUNDED BY ENTHUSIASTIC PEOPLE
DO THINGS RIGHT ... STRIVE FOR PERFECTION
THEN SIP FROM THE SWEET URN OF VICTORY**

The charisma, radiance, and energy displayed by enthusiastic persons bring sunshine to the lives of themselves and those around them. By utilizing the various lessons that follow, you too can easily make enthusiasm a part of your daily lifestyle. Early on, while learning to enhance your enthusiasm skills, it is common to feel awkward while performing various enthusiasm drills and exercises. Beginning enthusiasm learners can ease their initial clumsy feelings by approaching the learning of new attitude skills in a "fake it to make it" fashion.

The "fake it to make it" phase of enthusiasm development is perhaps the most exciting part of the enthusiasm learning process. When often repeated, "fake it to make it" exercises may create feelings of overkill. I remember that when I began using firm handshaking as an enthusiasm technique, my zestful and boisterous contacts with others caused them to feel uncomfortable and ill at ease. In time, I learned how to tone down my energetic gestures, and believe it or not, those who earlier were caught off guard by my "fake it to make it" actions began looking forward to our next chance to share my adapted greetings. This personal feedback assured me that my enthusiasm learning was alive, well, and getting better with each and every day.

Gestures of learned enthusiasm lead to the natural presence of greater self-confidence and the desire to demonstrate and share newly acquired skills with those you influence. Post–guided enthusiasm learning is at its best when integrated into daily actions at home, work, and in the community. At this point, you become a living model of the five E's (i.e., *E*xhibited *E*nthusiasm *E*ncourages *E*nhanced *E*xcellence). Continued presence and progressive use of the five E's allows one to reach higher levels of enthusiasm. The venture toward gaining 24-7 enthusiasm is a reality, in spite of those who feel it's impossible to be 100 percent positive all the time. In the later chapter "Remember 2B Positive," we will discuss how handmade motivational mementos aid in the achievement of eternal enthusiasm!

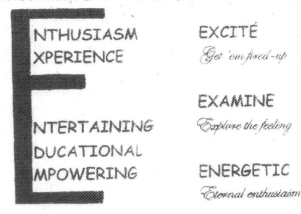

ENTHUSIASM ENCORAGES ENHANCED EXCELLENCE

NTHUSIASM
XPERIENCE

EXCITE
Get 'em fired-up

EXAMINE
Explore the feeling

NTERTAINING
DUCATIONAL
MPOWERING

ENERGETIC
Eternal enthusiasm

To improve your enthusiasm skills, begin to utilize Hubba Jubba's five tips for developing instant enthusiasm, which include (1) using I-2-I contact, (2) developing a firm and strong handshake, (3) saying your name proudly, (4) creating a hero-like signature, and (5) simply laffing more. A tremendous carryover for these tips is the natural ability to be enthusiastic, ensuring success in future career-related interviews, social interactions with others, and being a positive role model for children and other folks you are able to influence.

Hubba Jubba's Five Tips for Instant Enthusiasm

1. *Use I-2-I contact:* Eye contact is a major component for successful interviews, employment satisfaction, career advancement, and leadership pursuits. Many interviewers use eye contact as the first impression of those they visit. There is something about eye contact that communicates the presence of a strong, self-confident, and enthusiastic personality. Often persons prepare for interviews by referring to literature on successful interview strategies, and most of that literature speaks to the value of direct eye contact. More times than not, the pressure of an interview is such that eye contact gestures are forgotten until after the visit is over. Gazing into the eyes of another while conversing can be a distracting and frightful experience, but if one is comfortable with eye contact as a learned skill, he or she can employ this positive interview technique. An easy approach for learning eye contact habits is to avoid looking into another's eyes, instead focusing on his or her hairline while speaking with them. This takes some pressure off of having to use direct eye contact in the beginning. The one you are chatting with will think you are looking him or her in the eye, but really you're not. In time, you will become comfortable using the hairline option, and soon you will be able to move downward to actual I-2-I contact. Mastery of this enthusiasm skill

guarantees the possession of a most valuable and positive life skill.

2. *Give a firm handshake:* Another way to effectively transmit positive energy is through a firm and enthusiastic handshake. In the teen years of my life, my father often encouraged me to have my leather shoes shined when I wanted to make a positive impression. Now, some six decades later, shoe styles are so varied that the shoe shine concept is somewhat passé. Today, an alternate way to make a genuine first impression is by a firm handshake. Back in those old days, it was not fashionable for women to use handshakes as an act for greeting others. But today it is common for persons of all ages and genders to greet others with a handshake, even several times in the same day. When I began to advocate hearty handshakes, I was amazed to find out most folks are content to get by using only slight and limp hand greetings.

The first thing one must do when developing a more positive handshake is to squeeze another's hand in a sturdy fashion. If the hand you are shaking seems to be as excited with the contact as you are, then tighten the grip even more, and if they do the same, make the occasion even more delightful by putting both of your arms into the act. Such instances treat the shakers with meaningful and energetic moments of shared enthusiasm. When adding more dynamic efforts to your handshaking, make sure you never "outshake" persons who share limp and loose hand greetings. But when two strong handshakes meet each other, there is a resounding clash of thunder in the air, and mutual feelings of great joy and enthusiasm linger for a while.

Here is a special thought for women readers (or men with small hands), who wish to master this enthusiasm skill. Years ago when I attended a motivational sales seminar of all male participants, the idea of a strong handshake was featured as a symbol of power and control over potential clients and the opposite sex. Such actions fall short as an effort to convey personal enthusiasm. Most often a male's hand is considerably larger than a female's, so ladies are left in a defensive position and have limited opportunity to return personal positive hand gestures. Ah, but ladies, if you grasp another's hand from the middle knuckles down, squeeze hard, and add circular jump-rope-in-the-park or saw-the-log-in-the woods movements, you will experience the benefits of the aggressive handshake concept. So don't delay; begin using firm handshakes today!

3. *Say your name proudly:* Every person is born to be a star. We are all capable of being the best we can be at whatever we do; to do so is our birthright! To become the star you were meant to be, you must begin to act, look, and sound like one. What better way to share personal enthusiasm than by always saying your name proudly. The next time you hear a celebrity's name (whether a politician, athlete, or entertainer) announced on a public address system, pay attention to the volume and emotion in the voice of the introducer. By practicing ways to say your name with gusto and enthusiasm, you take a giant step toward becoming a drum major for enthusiasm!

4. *Create a hero signature:* Everyone should possess a hero signature! Successful people tend to have signatures with unusual and unique forms of "pen-person-ship." Most people scribe their name in a very clear and readable way. This makes sense, because it is necessary for owners of the signature to be identified, especially on tests and in other identity-related situations. A clever way to use your hero signature is to write a readable signature when needed, and then place your hero signature on top of it. If your positive karma is working at the time, maybe your hero signature will bring you bit of luck on the test (ha-ha!). So begin designing your exciting and enthusiastic hero signature today!

5. *Laff more:* The spirited healing, self-esteem building, and positive attitude development associated with hearty laffter is a stepping stone to higher levels of emotional maturity and enthusiasm mastery. The more times you use hearty laffter to ease stress, lessen anger, and combat adversity, the more healthy, happy, and successful you will be! So discover your best laff and share it ten seconds longer every day!

The Enthusiasm Its

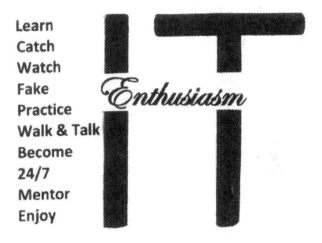

| Learn |
| Catch |
| Watch |
| Fake |
| Practice |
| Walk & Talk |
| Become |
| 24/7 |
| Mentor |
| Enjoy |

Here are ten actions related to the learning of enthusiasm skills:

1. *Learn it* through serious involvement with the knowledge and techniques for catching, learning, and sharing enthusiasm.
2. *Catch it* through a solid commitment to develop and apply the practical uses of enthusiasm-learning concepts.
3. *Watch it* by observing the sounds and moves used by persons who are already demonstrating enthusiastic gestures and attitudes.
4. *Fake it* by privately and publicly using pretend practice gestures (e.g., fake-it-to-make-it drills) to gain accelerated

learning of your enthusiasm-building skills. Executing these drills may seem a bit much early on, but doing so is a low-risk approach for achieving outside-the-box behaviors and attitudes of enthusiasm.

5. *Practice it* to overcome early feelings of shyness and uncomfortableness by using enthusiasm-building techniques on a daily basis, always remembering to fake it to make it. The more you fake it, the more comfortable you will become.

6. *Walk and talk it*, thereby orally and physically beginning to share your feelings of joy and enthusiasm with others. You know you are on the right track toward improved enthusiasm skills when your daily acquaintances begin asking if something is wrong with you because they can't quite put their finger on what's going on with you. Moreover, this marks the time in your enthusiasm learning when it is appropriate to start sharing the nature of your newfound enthusiasm with them.

7. *Become it* as you are able to feel the dawning of more and more personal enthusiasm within you. Each and every day finds you growing more eager to greet the excitement of tomorrow's sunrise.

8. *24-7 it*. Maturing to a full-time drum major for enthusiasm enables the mastery of positive human life skills and feelings of self-confidence, human success, and happiness;

9. *Mentor it* by sharing your investment in self-learned enthusiasm to organize individual and group enthusiasm experiences for your family, friends, and peers.

10. *Enjoy* it as those around you begin to recognize, admire, and inhale the positive and enthusiastic nature of your very presence. The power vested in these ventures empowers you with an endless supply of positive energy and inner satisfaction.

An allegiance to the use of these enthusiasm-building strategies should convince readers that enthusiasm can be taught and learned. However, this awareness is only the tip of the iceberg. Your progressive learning provides you with an option to commit to a higher level of enthusiasm mastery by sharing your developing talents with others. My passion for sharing enthusiasm is embraced by the lines I use at the end of my written correspondences: "Teaching others to love themselves is the greatest thrill of all" or "I mentor enthusiasm; so can you!"

The Enthusiasm–Laffter Connection

This idea began developing during my first six years as a high school teacher, coach, counselor, and animated sports official (1965–71), and in quite an unknowing manner. The concept has evolved to become the major passion impacting my current teaching, lecturing, and mentoring styles. Upon joining the physical education department faculty at the University of California San Diego (UCSD) in the fall of 1971, I thrived on the challenge, to use my classroom as a laboratory for creating, designing, and sharing exciting and entertaining educational experiences. First off, I began to incorporate visualization drills into my physical education classes, which surprisingly resulted in regular acceleration of beginning student tennis skills.

Secondly, I was able to design a course titled Psychology of Sports Officiating, which was intended to improve the skills of student intramural sport officials. This provided me quite an exciting outlet for extending my love of officiating, as I had just been axed from pursuits to become a Major League baseball umpire a few years earlier. The combination of my dynamic officiating gestures and visualization drills assisted students to quickly improve their officiating skills, not only for campus intramural sports but also for youth, high school, and college contests as well. During and since my years at UCSD, the student officials I taught have earned in excess of $3.5 million; dozens of them used year-round officiating to finance their entire college education, and many are still officiating today!

As the officiating class became more and more popular, students would often enroll in the course just to associate with the positive energy and enthusiasm it provided. At this point I began to broaden my enthusiasm-sharing skills across the campus community. My fond passion for offering Sharing of Enthusiasm presentations on campus, in the community, and at professional meetings aided in my regular receipt of faculty advancements and promotions.

And then—ta-da!—along came laffter. By complete chance, I bumped into research on the healing and pro-wellness uses of hearty laffter. And in less time than it took to explain it here, the enthusiasm–laffter connection was born. And I must admit, it has been very, very good to me.

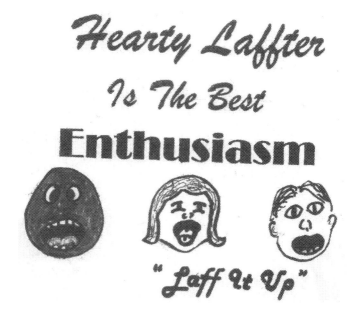

Chapter 2

There's Magic in Our Laffter

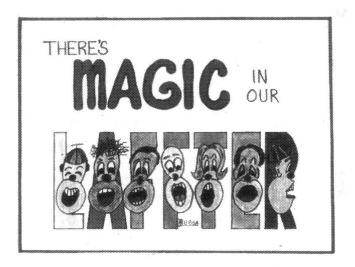

Ha ha ha! Yuk yuk yuk! Har har har! Oye oye oye! Arh arh arh! Yo yo yo! Ja ja ja! Eeeya eeya eeyaa! I love to laff; how about you? Laffter is good medicine. It's our grandest expression of joy and enthusiasm. It is infectious and contagious. Laffter is the universal symbol of goodwill, and most importantly, it's free; the cost is nothing!

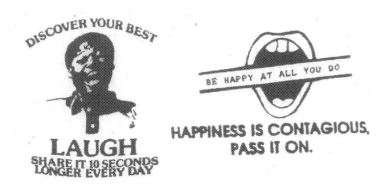

First of all, let's recognize that "gelotology" is the scientific name for the study and research of laffter. Hearty laffs are good for our health; they are spirit lifters and attention getters. They are sunshine on a cloudy day. They are high-level sources of energy, stress reducers, anger easers, and triggers for greater creativity. Hearty and healing laffter is a wide-open-mouthed action that causes air to pass over the vocal chords at sixty miles per hour. What does your best laff look like? What does it sound like? Discover it by laffing in your favorite mirror; then begin doing it ten seconds longer every day. In so doing, enable yourself to feel more enthusiastic and successful at all you do.

Recent research heralds the positive impact laffter has on our lives. Newspaper and magazine articles frequently discuss the topic, and many groups have been formed to promote the healing power of laffter in the workplace, at home, and within healing facilities. The therapeutic values of laffter include stress and anger reduction, lung workouts, body healing, immune system activation, easing of pain, presence of joy, enhanced self-esteem, and increased creativity. The content of this chapter differs from the popular approaches used by most facilitators of healthy laffter concepts. This added approach to the positive use of laffter goes beyond the reach of others by providing techniques for generating self-initiated responses of joy. Facilitators of traditional laffter therapy routines rely on such efforts as jokes, clowning, reading funny stories, and sharing cartoons and humorous videos.

The following discussion will focus on the anatomy of hearty laffter—what it looks and sounds like. In so doing, self-initiated efforts are presented to generate healthy laffter while eliminating the need for laffter learners to rely on others to provide healing laffs in their lives.

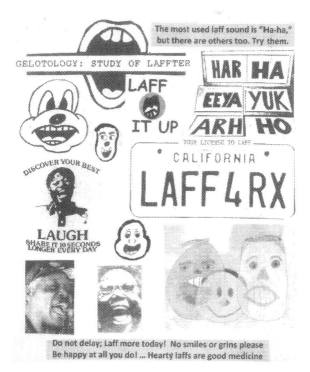

This alternate approach is a response to the following questions: What can I do when there is no one to tell me a joke? What do I do when my clown friends are not around? What happens if the batteries in my laffter box run out? What do I do when I'm not at home and there are no joke books or funny videos around? Those who can initiate their own laff sounds are able to jump-start actions needed to create the benefits of hearty laffter.

Let's Learn To Laff More

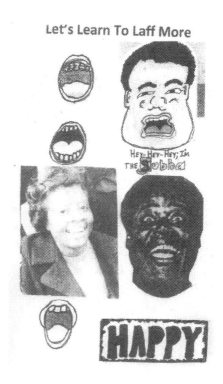

So what is a hearty laff? This is best answered by understanding what a hearty laff is not. Hearty laffter is a facial gesture unlike frowns, smiles, or grins. Smiling yellow cartoon faces have become a symbol of joy and fun, but smiles and grins lack the physical ability to access the benefits of hearty laffter. To prove this point, put a smile on your lips (keeping the lips together) and try to pass air over your vocal chords at sixty miles per hour and make hearty laff sounds; it can't be done. Now put on a grin (top teeth on lower lip) and attempt to make a hearty laff sound. Now how about that—it can't be done either. Smiles and grins lack the energy to allow healthy and healing laffter sounds to occur. However, when wide-open-mouth gestures are used, exposing the dark and deep areas in the rear of the mouth (as happens during a big yawn), loud and hearty laffter is available. In using such gestures, one is able to experience the magic of hearty laffter. To further understand this concept, place your hand on your throat while trying to create hearty laffter with a smile or grin. What did you feel? Now do the same thing while using a robust laff sound (like *yuk yuk yuk*), and you can actually feel air passing through your throat! Prolonged hearty laffter introduces chemicals (endorphins) into the blood and then initiates the various therapeutic benefits hearty laffter provides.

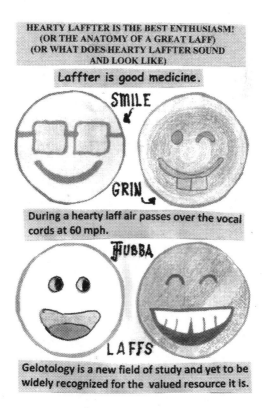

HEARTY LAFFTER IS THE BEST ENTHUSIASM!
(OR THE ANATOMY OF A GREAT LAFF)
(OR WHAT DOES HEARTY LAFFTER SOUND
AND LOOK LIKE)

Laffter is good medicine.

SMILE

GRIN

During a hearty laff air passes over the vocal cords at 60 mph.

HUBBA

LAFFS

Gelotology is a new field of study and yet to be widely recognized for the valued resource it is.

Hearty human laffter is the greatest expression of success and happiness; it is the outer gesture of inner self-confidence. When one is feeling great, laffter is automatically there. But when Old Person Fate deals from the bottom of the deck and the good times fade, laffs seem to vanish into thin air.

It is during these times of declining enthusiasm that self-initiated moments of laffter can reverse the ebbing tides of negative feelings. All you have to do is utilize any of the following actions:

1. Listen to ten minutes of prerecorded sounds of laffter on your cell phone or computer to restore yourself to a happy mood.
2. Call yourself on your cell phone and listen to your recorded voice message, featuring laffs galore, and then leave a laffter-filled message for yourself—and, of course, immediately play back the message.
3. Advertise the laffing images you have placed throughout your environment and view them to instantly regain a positive mental perspective.
4. Make a video recording on your "at the fingertips" technological equipment of a group participating in the game "ring of laffter." The group forms a standing circle and begins clapping their hands to the blare of danceable background music, and one by one each person advances to the center of the circle and then enthusiastically moves his or her hips to the beat of the music. Before departing to his or her original spot, each person sustains hearty laffter sounds and body gestures for a minimum of five seconds. Watching any part of the video of this game is guaranteed to rapidly replace clouds of despair with rays of warm and bright sunshine!

The most noted person to have influenced laffter research is the late Dr. Norman Cousins (1915–2000). He was a peace advocate, writer, and lecturer, as well as executive director of the *Saturday Review* (1940–78). He also served as a faculty member in the school of medicine at the University of California–Los Angeles. During the 1960s Cousins lay flat on his back with limited mobility because of a terminal affliction related to nerve failures in his spinal cord and an inability to sleep at night, due to a severe arthritic condition. Dismayed by constant pain, endless medications, and sleepless nights, he devised a holistic plan to reverse these devastating conditions. He moved out of the hospital and into a nearby hotel room with around-the-clock nursing service.

His health treatments included intravenous doses of vitamin C, rather than injections for his spinal cord issues. The continual drip of vitamin C into his body allowed him to maintain the doses in his system longer than by liquid injections which caused the rapid exit of the vitamins from his body. Laffing while viewing *Candid Camera* videos provided him with at least two hours of painless sleep, and when the pain returned, he simply viewed and laffed at the tapes to enjoy another two hours of pain-free sleep. The vitamin C process eliminated his spinal cord problems, while the laffter routines eventually relieved his arthritic discomfort. His amazing use of laffter as a healing procedure gained him worldwide recognition as the father of laffter research and led to his best-selling book entitled *The Anatomy of an Illness.*

In July 1984, Dr. Cousins gathered with a dozen of my UC San Diego students to discuss the matters related to his remarkable healing experiences. Not only were his tales of humor healing a delight to everyone in the audience, but the more proactive students were especially excited when the discussion shifted to world politics and peace solutions. This special gathering took place in the offices of the late Joan Kroc, whose philanthropic resources were sponsoring Dr. Cousins's research at the UCLA medical center. When the conversation reached the point of controversy, a rather conservative Kroc aide signaled for a shift in the line of conversation. However, being the down-to-earth person he was, Dr. Cousins ignored the gesture and continued sharing his thoughts on the need for peace in Vietnam. At the time of this meeting, the student protest movement was in full swing on college campuses across the nation, and student participants had the opportunity to be a part of a once-in-a-lifetime learning experience with a relevant worldwide change agent!

Hearty Laffter Tips

Tips for Hearty Laffers

      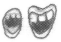

In order to build a lasting allegiance to the use of hearty laffter and its resulting benefits, begin using any of the following laffter tips:

1. Every morning, give five big laffs in the mirror while grooming for the day.
2. Deck your walls and hallways with laffing images of yourself, your family, and others.
3. Observe, enjoy, and congratulate the great laffs shared by others.
4. When you hear new and creative laffs, take time to spell them out.
5. Try on for size the great laffs you observe; maybe they will fit you.
6. For variety, alter your laff sounds and face gestures from time to time.
7. Record five minutes of laffs by yourself and others to play back when your spirits need a lift.
8. Outlaff the laffs others give when they are laffing at you during embarrassing moments.
9. Place any number of various laff sounds on your phone.
10. Film the fondest laffs you observe each day.
11. Regularly take laffing selfies to capture the best laffs of your day.

12. When around moody persons, laff loud and long till they laff too.
13. Create group posters and collages exhibiting wild laffs by all.
14. Remind family and friends that smiles and grins are not healthy laffs.
15. Use laffter flash cards, causing others to laff with you.
16. Test the state of your current laffs by regularly evaluating them in the mirrors of your life.
17. During idle moments (when otherwise daydreaming), occupy yourself by doodling creative and jolly images of laffter.
18. Tell a funny tale about an experience you had with a person, during his or her celebration-of-life service.
19. Whenever your day needs a lift, LAFF IT UP!
20. Make the world your laboratory for developing and sustaining high levels of laffter and enthusiasm.

There are times when hearty laffter can be labeled as inappropriate behavior. Laffter should never be used to ridicule or degrade another person. Many facilitators of grieving skills encourage mourners to recall their happiest memories of a deceased one and then use these thoughts to momentarily break the sorrow looming in the air. If you feel like doing so, recall a funny experience you had with the deceased and share it at his or her funeral service. How sad it is when the homecoming services for persons who routinely shared loads of happiness with others are laid to rest without any references to the joy they shared.

Think happy, act happy, and you will be happy. A good way to achieve this end is to wear apparel advertising the happy faces of you, friends, relatives, and others. This can be done by sharing images of self-joy (laffing selfies) on T-shirts, caps, sweatshirts, drinking mugs and glasses, jackets, group apparel, and so many more things. What an exciting thought: wearing and sharing joy and happiness!

A rather interesting idea I share with myself is identifying a list of those I have known and another of others who impressed me with their extreme passion for sharing hearty laffter. I encourage you to create a similar list of the heartiest laffers you have seen, and to go so far as to design a collage featuring their faces of great joy. Of course, making a laffing collage of yourself is not a bad idea either!

Best Laffs by Friends	Best Laffs by Celebrities
Harold Addison Sr.	Louis Armstrong
Emmett Ashford	Lucille Ball
Betsy Cemone	Joe E. Brown
Len Burnett	Carol Burnett
Aunt Fannie Lee Mason	Magic Johnson
Leo Dejon	Phyllis Diller
Sabrina Kinder	Moms Mobley
Donna Kumara	Willie Mays
Barbara Stone	Goose Tatum
Phil Raphael	Dionne Warwick
Clancy Davis	Red Skelton

Another way to share hearty laffter with others is to create words to sing along to your favorite upbeat tunes. These happy actions provide moments of uninterrupted laffter sounds at family get-togethers, social gatherings, and classroom and workplace oral presentations. Professional speakers often begin their speaking engagements with a joke because it relaxes the audience and encourages them to better receive the information to be shared. When using this technique, I sing my Hubba Jubba songs line by line, having the audience repeat after me; then, at the end of each verse, I use my laffter flash cards (reading "Ha ha!" "Yuk yuk!" "Oye oye!" "Har har!" etc.) to initiate several moments of hearty and healthy laffter. The activity has even greater impact when I walk down the aisles sharing animated belly laffs. One of the songs is called "Have a Happy-Happy Day" and is sung to the tune of "Happy Days Are Here Again."

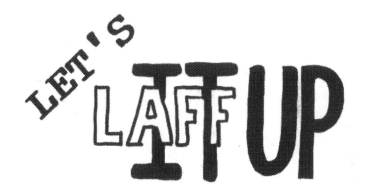

Verse #1

Have a happy day today

Have a happy-happy day today

Make everything go your way

Have a happy-happy day (Laffter flash cards)

Verse #2

Happy days for me and you

Happy-happy days for me and you;

Let's be enthused at all we do

Happy days for me and you (Laffter flash cards)

For best results, repeat the verses a second time.

Another "get 'em laffing" song is Hubba's "Laff It Up." The tune for this song is from "If You're Happy and You Know It." Each time I say "laff it up," the groups raises the roof (raising both arms, palms to the ceiling) and repeats any of the laffter flash cards two times (e.g., "laff it up, yuk yuk! Laff it up, yuk yuk!*). Most often I use this song as the closing activity of a Hubba Jubba presentations.

"Hubba's Laff It Up Song"

Laff it up (har-har); Laff it up (har-har); Laff it up (har-har); When your day needs a lift laff it up (har-har); When your day needs a lift laff it up (har-har); When your day is stressed and bad and you're feeling mad and sad; When your day needs a lift laff it up (har-har); when your day needs a lift laff it up (har-har).

21

Perhaps a place where some people would not expect to find laffter is in their halls of worship. Pulpit speakers commonly use humorous remarks while delivering messages to their flocks. There are several scriptures in The Bible referencing joy and laffter; these include Genesis 17:17; Genesis 18:12; Genesis 21:6; Proverbs 17:22; Proverbs 31:25; Psalm 59:8; Psalm 126:1–2; Ecclesiastes 3:4; and Luke 6:21.

It must also be noted that while some clergy refer to Biblical references on joy and laffter, others make the point that there is no connection between laffter and holy joy. Feel free to search the Internet for "Biblical Joy and Laughter" to get a closer look at this controversy.

The varied uses of hearty laffter as healing tools are obvious. Focus on laffter as a positive health experience is becoming more and more popular every day. Once again, the uniqueness of these pages on the positive uses of laffter lies in the fact that outside influences are not necessary to unleash the healing powers of hearty laffter. Once you understand the anatomy of hearty laffter, and its many benefits, all you have to do to experience the fruits of hearty laffter is employ repeated actions of sending air over the vocal chords at sixty miles per hour. The values of hearty laffter beckon us; the high tides of joviality are with us; let us put our ships of hearty laffter to sea!

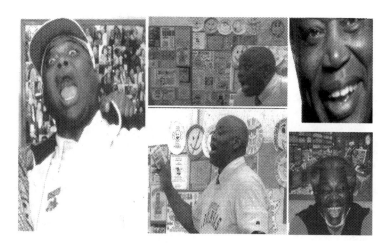

Chapter 3

Creativity Is Me and You Too

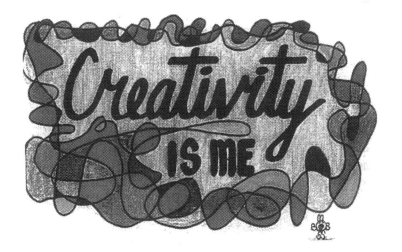

Human creativity is the crowning jewel for developing the mind's potential. Exploring even the smallest segment of our imagination allows us to tap the vast limits of our creative talents. So don't delay, begin developing your mind more today! When we train our minds to create images of our future goals, we are able to achieve higher levels of self-esteem, success, and happiness.

To be the best you can be, you must improve your talents a bit more every day. Just showing up to practice every day is not enough. Using pretend practice drills will provide you with the added reps needed to accelerate the level of your playing skills. Don't delay, become an imagery freak today!

Early in my teaching career I discovered I had a natural knack for changing creative thoughts into useful concepts and images. A logical reason for this talent goes back to the art minor I earned during my undergraduate studies. When I gained a faculty position at UC San Diego, my creativity came full cycle as a result of the creative challenges made available through faculty opportunities to research and develop improved teaching techniques. Also, my allegiance to mental imagery (pretend practice) instruction techniques enabled me to focus on imagination-expanding classroom experiences and urge students to recognize that creativity is me and them too!

Here are a few ways to improve your creativity: doodle images of your positive thoughts and feelings, explore a variety of body and facial gestures (laffs) before the favorite mirror of your life, keep a daily journal nearby to note the thoughts and hunches crossing your mind during the day and while sleeping at night, perform pretend practice drills to act out your new motions and gestures of enthusiasm, and utilize current technological resources to view pretend practice activities. By utilizing these suggested actions along with others created on your own, you can achieve a mastery of greater creativity!

At this point, it is appropriate to mention the importance of visual aids in developing and sharing positive-attitude-development concepts. These visual items serve not only as motivation for users but also as tools for sharing later enthusiasm-building ideas with others. Two of my favorite visual teaching images are the Moss-Cess Success Profile and the Moss-Cess Success Process. Both of these items were created early in my teaching career (1973 and 1974).

Over the years, they have served as class handouts, wall posters, and framed gifts rewarding outstanding achievements by my students, family members, and friends. The history of the Moss-Cess Success Profile stems from a presentation I attended by the noted motivation guru Earl Nightingale. Following his lecture, I was inspired to create visual images to better share the self-motivation ideas presented to those I influence. At the time, I was working on a master's degree in counselor education and experiencing the dawning of African American heritage awareness. By wearing an African American hairstyle, I was able to, for the first time in my life, openly display personal pride in my ethnic identity. While my class peers could not understand why I would want to promote an Afro hair style, I basked in the wisdom gained by finally sharing something in an academic setting that looked like me! I have since encouraged others to create their own personal profiles as self-motivational tools enabling them to experience greater feelings of self-esteem. I must note that the Moss-Cess Success Profile maintains the exact same significance today as it did when it was created in 1973.

Components of the Moss-Cess Profile

The seven items on the Moss-Cess Success Profile are guidelines for the progressive development of an enthusiasm-oriented lifestyle. Upon reviewing the profile's individual units, it is important to ponder the contents for your own success chart or profile.

The Moss-Cess Success Profile

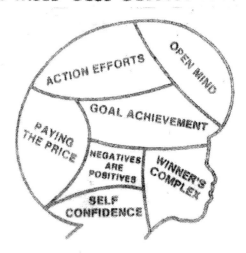

SELF CONFIDENCE: Knowledge of, and faith in ones personal ability to achieve individual success; Every person should boast: "I am the greatest in my field!"

GOAL ACHIEVEMENT: An organized and pre-determined plan developing a strong commitment for turning thoughts into things; Success is a journey, never a destination.

OPEN MIND: A constant quest for new knowledge and self awareness, in order to effectively stimulate creativity and human potential growth; Knowledge is truth and power.

NEGATIVES ARE POSITIVES: Recognizing that out of failure and adversity, seeds of something greater are planted; Success blooms from failure.

WINNER'S COMPLEX: A burning desire to pursue the unlimited nature of the human success mechanism; Every man and woman is born to succeed.

PAYING THE PRICE: Nothing is achieved in the absence of persistence and determination; Success comes before work only in the dictionary.

ACTION EFFORTS: A blending of the above items, to yield a mastery of the "I'm gonna" attitude, leading to a higher level of creative maturity; The "I did it" complex.

• *Self-Confidence:* This is the knowledge of and faith in one's personal ability to achieve individual success; every person should boast: "I am the greatest in my field!" Always remember that loving yourself is the greatest thrill of all. Through the use of the enthusiasm-sharing concept, one is able to promote the positive body language and verbal responses symbolic of such lifestyle skills as stress control, anger management, leadership initiative, and positive relations with others.

- *Goal Achievement:* Organized goals with predetermined plans to develop them into a strong commitment for turning thoughts into things are a grand key for achieving personal success. Success is a journey, never a destination. One's personal goals need not be realistic or to the liking of others; they only need to be firmly embedded in the mind and actions of the pursuer.

- *Open Mind:* This requires a constant quest for new knowledge and awareness in order to effectively stimulate creativity and human potential for growth. Knowledge is truth and power. An open mind is always seeking new ideas and approaches for improving life for itself and others. This guideline is also noted by a desire to expand one's knowledge on any number of topics, ask questions, and become a better listener.

- *Negatives are Positives:* While positive results are always desired, we must be ready to rebound from the failures, adversity, and disappointments challenging us along our highways to future success. It is important to learn from previous mistakes and, if at all possible, avoid repeating them again. We must maintain strength and focus within ourselves and control our emotions and attitudes when our success train may encounter temporary sidetracking. How do you look when you are upset, stressed-out, or angry? Become aware of your body gestures during both good and bad times, and begin training yourself to avoid looks of frustration and despair in adverse situations. Acquire the ability to look for and expect the best from yourself and others.

- W*inner's Complex:* This is a burning desire to pursue the unlimited nature of your human success mechanism and become the best person you can possibly be. Study and

> emulate the styles and gestures of those you know who are already achieving high levels of success.
>
> - *Paying the Price:* A common fact of life is that the worthiest things we want will often not be achieved in the absence of persistence, determination, and hard work. Figure out the things in life you enjoy doing the most, and become more involved with them. Investigate ways in which you might be able to turn any of them into part- or full-time money-making adventures. And lastly, learn to have more patience with yourself. Always remember, neither Rome nor Las Vegas was built in a day; the same is true of Timbuktu and Green Bay. And never forget your old friend ... what's his name? Oh yes, Ruddy Gazoodie, the guy no one can remember. Why? Because he refused to pay the price. Yuk yuk yuk!
> - *Action Efforts:* We are all born to become stars and be the greatest we can be. Establish daily entries in a diary or journal; post photos, posters, and collages across the walls of your living environment; make sure all these images reflect positive past events and the future amazing goals you desire to achieve. These efforts will cause a blending of the above items to yield a mastery of the "I'm gonna" attitude, leading to a higher level of creative maturity, the "I did it" complex.

The Moss-Cess Success Process

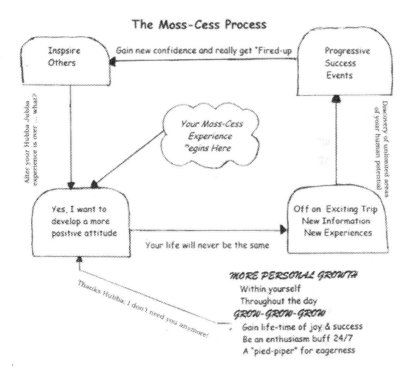

This image was born as a hastily created visual aid for a sports officiating class lecture back in 1974. The original diagram was put together in less than ten minutes, and the four corners were actually bases on a baseball field. Over the years, the process was updated from a sports focus to a success road map for audiences in general. It has served as a visual motivation guide encouraging lifestyle enrichment, and I've always encouraged those I influence to someday create their own success road map to inspire themselves and others. In so doing, many have been moved to say, "Hubba, thanks a lot for enhancing my enthusiasm skills, but I don't need you anymore!" How unique is that?

The process encourages users to expand their individual creativity by combining their thoughts and images in the form of personal efforts leading to their increased joy and enthusiasm. To begin the process, one must say, "Yes, I want to achieve greater enthusiasm, joy, and positive attitudes" (home plate). At this point, his or her life will never be the same.

Throughout the process, patrons receive learning from exciting, entertaining involvement facilitated by Hubba Jubba. These activities include such things as audiovisual aids, mini-lectures, songs, handmade motivation mementos, role-playing sessions, visualization (pretend) drills, and responses to brief quiz items. The content of *The Enthusiasm–Laffter Connection* is nothing more than a Hubba Jubba learning experience in writing. Most importantly, be it through an actual one-day workshop or reading the chapters of this book, learners are able to involve themselves with knowledge and labors of extreme enthuuuuusiasm!

As the process continues, participants are able to move on toward gaining progressive success experiences (first base) by discovering areas of their unlimited human potential. New enthusiasm buffs are urged to immediately weave learned experiences into their daily activities at home, work, school, and elsewhere. It is important at this time for positive-attitude-enrichment seekers to understand and then utilize the "fake it to make it" concept. Faking it is a key tool for maintaining the grit needed to ward off shyness, fear, hesitation, and doubt associated with trying something for the first time. It provides the mental toughness needed to stay on track when the tides of meekness and embarrassment creep ashore.

The onset of progressive success experiences (second base) allows one to gain a more confident outlook on life and really get "turned on"! Contrary to what many may think, a person *can* eventually develop and maintain an eternal attitude of enthusiasm on a 24-7 basis. As one begins to demonstrate the sunshine of enthusiasm on a consistent basis, even amid the dampness of rain, sleet, or snow, those closest to him or her will begin admiring what they once thought was behavior leading to future residency on the funny farm. The zestful conduct previously causing confusion and conflict now fosters comments of admiration and appreciation!

The natural nature of the process leads to its protégé inspiring others as he or she rounds third base, heading for home. As the cycle completes its course with the Moss-Cess Success Process, the now complete enthusiasm sharer crosses home plate and returns to the sidelines to organize his or her own personal options for future use. Through workplace and community leadership involvement, the new mentors can now test the quality of their developing wings for sharing joy and enthusiasm.

During the time immediately following completion of the process, it is important for recently crowned enthusiasm mentors to design and develop effective materials to assist them in their future roles as facilitators of eternal enthusiasm-learning experiences. Moreover, the spirit of creativity must always be present as they begin sharing their personalized ventures as pied pipers for positive attitude instruction. It is time for them to say, "Thanks Hubba; I don't need you anymore!"

Chapter 4

Remembering 2B Positive

Always Remember

2 - B Positive

Up to this point, you have been able to observe several creative ways to add more enthusiasm to your daily lifestyle. Here is a quick glance at a number of these items: enthusiasm-teaching concepts, the laffter-enthusiasm connection, anatomy of hearty laffs, easy-to-use laffter tips, the recognition that creativity is me and you too, and the Moss-Cess Success Profile and Success Process.

Now it's time to examine a most innovative and valuable concept—remembering 2B positive. When joy and confidence are on our plates, there is no need to remember how to maintain the moment. However, when fate deals from the bottom of the deck and our enthusiasm begins to fade, how can we keep the good feelings rolling? Most times folks rely on willpower, spiritual values, or good luck to rescue sinking positive attitudes. Remembering 2B positive is a backup strategy allowing a variety of ways to encourage extended happiness and confident moments during times of adversity. Call them "ways to provide positive attitudes 24-7," or "eternal enthusiasm." These hand-crafted motivation memento items include stickers, happy faces on paper plates, posters and collages, bookmarks, journal entries, audiovisual aids, greeting cards, and any other efforts to create personal environments with positive images. These mementos can be found in such resources as photos (half of them of you), news clippings, magazine articles, drawings, websites, and clip art.

Stickers

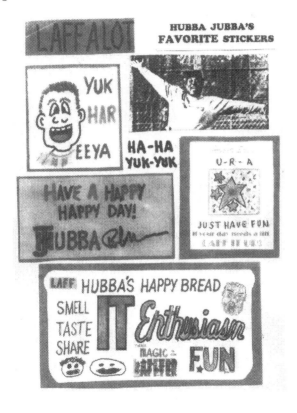

The sticker concept was born in the mid-1990s when I became an elementary school physical education teacher with the San Diego School District. One of the first things that caught my eye were the stickers teachers use as tools for encouraging and rewarding positive student behavior. Because I was a legend in my own mind and modesty has never been one of my virtues, I created Hubba Jubba stickers to reward students exhibiting academic success and good behavior. The stickers, with their happy images and motivational messages, gained instant success with students and adults alike. In less time than it took to explain, I began to use the stickers as "remember 2B positive" mementos for participants attending my public lectures, professional presentations, and in-service activities.

The simple instructions for making personalized motivation stickers are as follows:

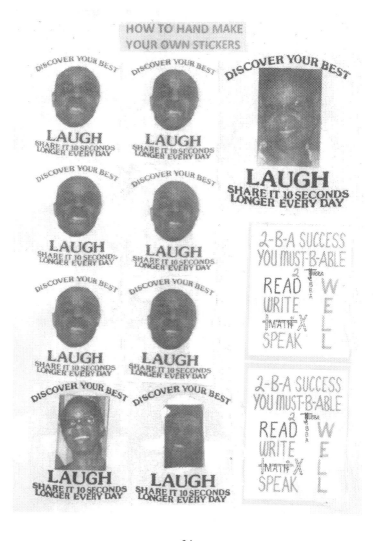

1. Create a desired sticker image on an 8½" × 11" sheet of paper.
2. Scan it into a computer.
3. Using the multiple-image tool, create at least eight images on a page; I normally put nine on a page.
4. Copy your image onto full-sized sheets of shipping label paper.
5. Cut the stickers out.
6. Pass out the personalized stickers to family, friends, and others, and in so doing, enjoy the thrill of sharing your enthusiasm!

Note: Placing four images on your label paper provides giant economy-size stickers for selected special recipients.

Greeting Cards

While the use of stickers is still fresh in our minds, let's discuss making greeting cards as an excellent extended follow-up application of the sticker concept. I first made greeting cards after reading about a high school on the East Coast that earned thousands of dollars selling student-made Christmas cards. At the time, I thrived on sharing my classroom enthusiasm at a secondary charter school providing U-Turn learning options for at-risk students (in fact, the school was named YOU School). While assigned as an art teacher and ASB advisor, I considered how neat it would be to have the art students make the cards and have the ASB students market them as a school fund-raising project. The activity was only a modest success (it earned only $150), but I stored the idea in the back of my mind for future use.

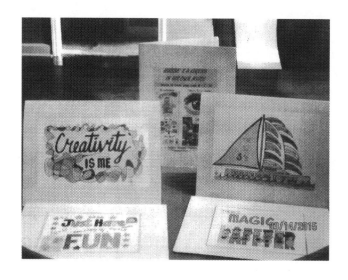

So now let's fast-forward some ten (Add "five") years, to the year 2000. I had gained popularity as a "pied piper of stickers" while teaching physical education at two elementary schools. On one bright and sunny day, the thought struck me to triple the size of Hubba Jubba stickers, place them on one half of folded sheets of 8½" × 11" card stock, and send them to folks as friendship greeting cards. This has been quite a rewarding venture for me; can it be one for you too?

Happy Paper Plate Faces Galore

Positive attitudes are encouraged when positive images are placed throughout the environments we encounter day in and day out. The presence of laffing faces (remember, no smiles or grins) can remind us to remain upbeat amid times of frustration and adversity. A very popular activity I use during my motivational presentations involves participants drawing happy faces on paper plates. The completed happy images are suitable for attachment on the family refrigerator, hallways, and bedroom walls. When preparing happy paper plate faces, be sure to use uncoated paper plates so that colored pencils, pens, crayons, and markers will easily adhere to plate surfaces. Before any colors are used, the activity facilitator should review the faces after participants have lightly penciled their faces on the plates, making sure each face covers the entire plate bottom and includes a mouth that is wide open in laffter. When finished, all of the plate surfaces should be completely colored in, including the outer ridges.

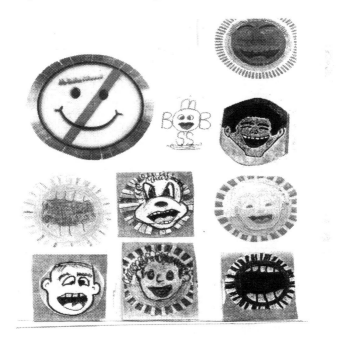

To further celebrate happy faces, one can mount multiple laffing faces of himself or herself, or family and friends, on colored card stock. One more option is to engage folks attending seminars, birthday parties, or other social gatherings in an opening activity of drawing happy faces on small paper plates, taping a loop of yarn on the back of the plate, placing their names somewhere on the plates, and then wearing the plates around their necks as unique and happy name tags.

Bookmarks

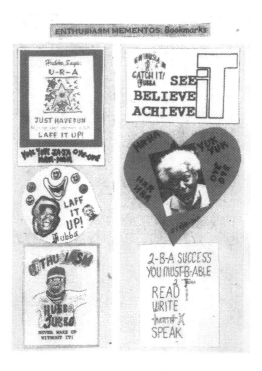

This is a worthy idea for promoting classroom and home literacy experiences. The activity simply encourages the positive feelings gained from using personal bookmarks as a part of student reading efforts. Handmade bookmarks can also be used as group fund-raising projects or simply passed on as gifts to friends and family members.

Posters and Collages

These items include any positive images reminding us to remember to be positive at all times, especially when there is an absence of good things going on. Posters and collages are made up of such items as past and present photos, favorite thoughts, religious sayings, happy faces, slogans, and anything else striking a positive note when negative conditions begin to prevail.

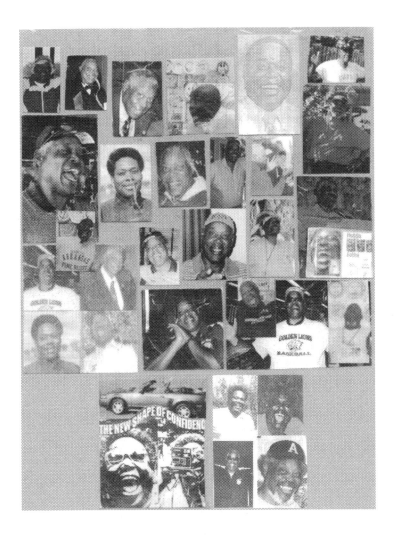

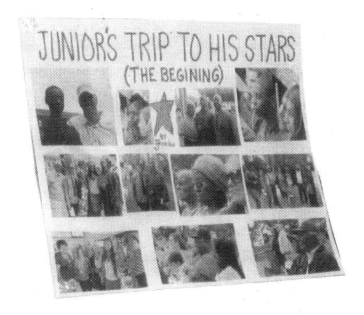

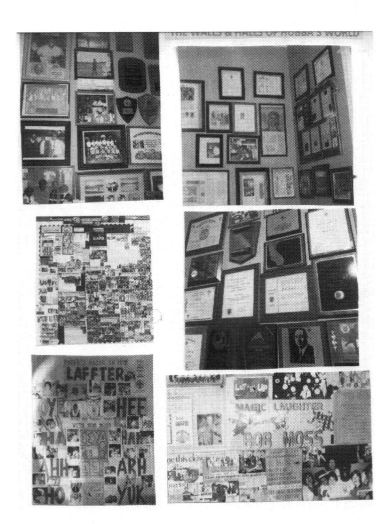

Poetry and Other Readings

The poems, slogans, and spiritual references capable of energizing your personal pursuits should be close to your hand at all times. Perhaps the best use of these items is achieved when they are written by you or someone you know.

Audiovisual Aids

In the fast-paced technological world we live in today, it goes without saying that most everyone carries a cell phone. In this age, audiovisual resources linger only an arm's length away from us. Through the wonders of cellular devices, we have the ability to store any of the "remember 2B positive" techniques and immediately access them to maintain or regain positive thoughts and gestures.

The routine habit of creating handmade "remember 2B positive" mementos is a valuable resources for aiding in the 24-7 presence of joy and enthusiasm. Which of the "remember 2-B positive" mementos will you create first?

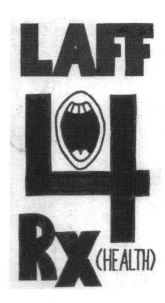

Chapter 5

The Twelve S's for Success

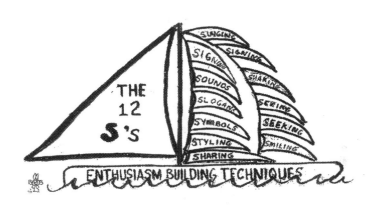

Every person is born with the potential to become a star! Stars shine, sparkle, glow, perform feats of excellence, and lead the way through darkness. How to discover and achieve lifelong feelings of stardom is what the pages of this book are all about. Why do so many folks fear being a star and avoid the desire to become one? If standing out from the crowd has never been a goal for you, why not try it on for size to see if it fits you? If you test-drive starlike actions and don't like them, then toss them out and continue merrily on your way. For those who feel a spark of positive energy when acting like a star, new feelings of empowerment and happiness are just around the corner!

In the beginning, one must fake it to make it. The process for awakening the stardom within you starts with the following actions:

1. Create a list of ten persons—five you've met through media resources and five from your actual daily life experiences—whom you believe are the most dynamic persons you know.
2. Study the voice tones, gestures, and spirits of those on your list.
3. Rehearse their styles with daily pretend practice exercises by gesturing, talking, and posing like them in front of mirrors.
4. Use your imagination to design a variety of handmade mementos, and place them throughout your environment.
5. Bask in the glory of the joy, confidence, and excitement your were born to experience!

Modesty has never been one of my virtues, so I'm sharing the examples below as a guide to kick-start the creation of your personal starlike images.

The twelve S's are a dozen words beginning with the letter *S* that identify simple and easy options for becoming a star by gaining and maintaining eternal enthusiasm and self-confidence. These items are valuable environmental management resources in tune with the previously discussed "remember 2B positive" concept.

Signs

Signs are enthusiasm illustrated. Deck your walls and hallways with positive images of yourself and others. The themes and scope of these images are limited only by your imagination and creativity. These signs can be in the form of framed photos or artwork. Ideal spots for positive signs can be on the wall directly beyond the threshold of your home and on its ceilings, walls, and bathroom mirrors.

Slogans

Slogans are a dime a dozen. Celebrate and refer to inspirational quotes written by others and you too. They can be in the form of poetry, scriptures, one-liners, or personal thoughts. While effective slogans abound, the best are those created by you! Following are a few examples of the original slogans I frequently use:

- For many a win and never a loss, treat yourself to an experience with Bob Moss.
- If your day needs a lift, laff it up!
- Hubba Jubba is my name; mentoring enthusiasm is my game.
- I'm the sunshine of my world; the length of my season shall be determined by the depths of my eternal enthusiasm.

Symbols

Symbols are images of the real you. Surround yourself with positive things. What do you feel like while in complete control of your day? What animals, nature forms, or man-made inventions do you best associate with your greatest moments of joy and enthusiasm? Place them across your environment to energize positive thoughts of yourself at all times. Whatever animal one may choose, it must be remembered that there is no such thing as a poor symbol. Lions and eagles are just as dynamic as frogs and turtles; it's all in the eye of the person involved. When one is at the top of his or her day, he or she may feel as sturdy as the mighty pyramids or as powerful as a beautiful waterfall.

Sounds

What you say is what you are. Sounds include the music you choose to listen and snap your fingers to. Oftentimes, many popular tunes seem to describe negative and lonely circumstances, such as encounters with lonely places like "heartbreak hotel."

Make sure the music you enjoy and snap your fingers to reflects positive moods and thoughts. Sounds also include the words from your lips and those of others around you. Positive self-talk and conversation with others are simply matters of choice. Enthusiasm sharers select music and words associated with positive thoughts and innuendos. A unique exercise for promoting the positive use of sounds is to organize a series of creative audio or video recordings featuring upbeat verbal thoughts, hearty laffter, inspirational readings, and peer conversations.

Shaking

A strong and firm handshake leaves a fine impression on those we meet and greet. This technique is based upon the idea that positive personal attitudes can be transmitted by physical contact, in the same way as the noncontact effects of eye-to-eye contact. The style of your handshake goes a long way toward determining the first impression others will have of you.

Styling

Work your moves and moods. We're all born to be a star; you can become a star by simply learning how to feel comfortable standing out in the crowd and become a more positive influence for your family, friends, coworkers, and others. By examining video recordings and mirror images of yourself using any variety of gestures similar to those used by models on runways, you can enhance your feelings of self-esteem. Make it a regular practice to develop your own forms of styling by pretending to walk and talk like the favorite stars in your life.

While video replay is a worthy feedback tool for viewing desired movements and moods, mirror reflections are the easiest and most convenient way to explore and improve alternate styling options. At first, practicing styling gestures may not come easily. Most often folks rarely observe their images for anything other than brushing teeth, combing hair, and generally preparing for public view. Using mirror reflections to style new images can be embarrassing and quite scary for those who have never used the technique before. But as with any other new activity, after repeated performances, what was once uncomfortable soon becomes a routine action.

Signing

Scribe your name with gusto. Create and use a "hero signature" as another practice for gaining the confidence and esteem demonstrated by your favorite stars and the successful persons you know. How many times a day do you sign your name? Is your signature any different today from what it was ten years ago? Would you have ever thought the manner in which you scribed your name would have anything to do with enhancing your personal enthusiasm? Learning to use an enthusiastic signature is just another way of developing greater personal enthusiasm and confidence.

Examine the handwriting style of any of the autographs you have received from famous and successful persons, and notice how they look. Persons who have to sign hundreds of autographs in a short period of time create signatures exhibiting unique enthusiastic qualities. So immediately begin to design and use your own hero signature!

Singing

Songs of triumph—everyone has one, two, or three. Identify favorite upbeat tunes and then sing or hum them throughout your day. Some people will prefer upbeat and lively tunes, while others will prefer softer or smoother sounds. The styles of these songs fit the fancy of the individual involved. These songs serve to celebrate the good times and provide a source of inspiration during times of stress and conflict. Everyone enjoys songs sung by their favorite crooners, but many hesitate to sing aloud in public because their voices are untrained. A great way for persons wanting to overcome shyness and gain greater self-confidence is for them to sing favorite theme songs, hymns, and oldies but goodies to themselves. Once one becomes comfortable singing aloud, he or she can make the choice of communicating positive thoughts by singing songs to others.

- Sing to mentally prepare for important personal events.
- Sing to bring sunshine to cloudy days.
- Sing to emphasize the main message during oral presentations.
- Sing to brighten gloomy group environments.
- Sing to inspire others dealing with frustrations, adversity, bad luck, or personal hardships.
- Sing to upgrade environments at family and social gatherings.
- Sing to simply maintain a high quality of eternal enthusiasm during every hour of every day.

Seeing

Observe grand gestures by others. This involves viewing the positive gestures of enthusiasm being used by others. While it is important to style your own gestures of enthusiasm, as mentioned earlier, it is important to observe the movements and moods of others too. By reviewing the styles of others, you are able to better design patterns for your own future enthusiasm profiles. The "seeing" technique requires you to examine possible enthusiasm moves and mood options by viewing mirror or window reflections and video recordings.

The study of body language is a growing field of research focusing on the manner in which our bodies move and how those movements can be interpreted. By utilizing "seeing" resources, we are able to watch and read the movements of others, and then design personal enthusiasm gestures to meet our own needs.

Seeking

Get a bit better every day. This idea includes the use of library and Internet resources to discover the knowledge you need to improve your life passions and gain more joy and enthusiasm. Seeking includes continued research, reading, and the questioning of pathways followed by those who have already reached the lofty goals you have set for yourself. Progressive development of our maximum human potential is dependent on keeping in touch with the latest ideas and techniques related to your fields of interest. Too many people fail to pursue continued learning, and deny any upper mobility for their professional and personal achievements. Therefore, it is important to gain daily knowledge. With today's technological resources, all you have to do is simply let your fingers to do the seeking.

Smiling

Promote hearty laffter. Remember, smiles and grins make us feel good, but it's only hearty laffs that can make us feel better and provide healthy and healing conditions.

Sharing

Sharing is the greatest S of all. What our world needs now is more enthusiasm sharing. My decades of teaching and modeling positive human gestures have led me to believe that teaching others to love themselves, through enthusiasm instruction, is the grandest thrill of all. The sharing of enthusiasm is both a conscious and unconscious occurrence. It is shared as I greet and meet others; facilitate classroom, in-service, and community presentations; and introduce folks to my garage walls, walk them through the halls of my home, and encourage them to create their own handmade mementos to share their own enthusiasm.

Of course, the book you are reading serves as my ultimate tool for sharing enthusiasm with you and others. The sharing of enthusiasm provides yet another approach for teaching enthusiasm. A popular thought I have always shared with my circle of peers is that we gain greater personal and professional growth through our efforts to inspire greatness in others. The plain and simple fact is that by firing up others, we are better able to fire ourselves up. As valuable a tool as the twelve S's are, their most meaningful use occurs when users exercise their individual creativity in applying any of the twelve S's. So off you go into exciting and satisfying adventures, sharing your enthusiasm instruction skills with others!

Chapter 6

Creative Visualization

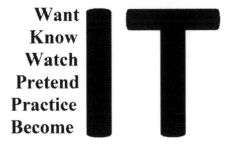

Creative Visualization
Mental Imagery
Pretend (Fake) Practice

Want
Know
Watch
Pretend
Practice
Become

While each of the previous topics has been a joy to explore, visualization (pretend practice) is one of my fondest of them all. Little did I know that adding it to the curricula of my UC San Diego physical education courses (back in 1972) would have a tremendous impact on most things I now do four decades later. Thanks to the outstanding use of visualization techniques (oftentimes referred to as mental imagery, pretend practice, or "faking it to make it" drills) as referenced by Maltz, Longino, Kryder, Frederick, Just, and Flynn (see more about their work on the later list of relevant resources), I was able to design and implement exciting ways to accelerate student learning of motor skills and personal attitudes.

Pretend practice is based upon the fact the human brain cannot tell the difference between an actual successful event and one vividly imagined. The act of imagination practice requires one to listen to recorded rhythms, view movements in front of mirrors, watch videotaped feedback, and imagine performances on the TV screen in his or her mind of doing actions correctly. Once one becomes aware of how to do a particular skill properly, he or she must go before a mirror and get the image of how it looks to perform the action correctly. At first the feel for the activity will seem awkward at best, but with more and more pretend repetitions, the task becomes more comfortable. Once one has gained the feeling of doing it right, he or she is ready to gain even more repetitions by repeating them during their daily adventures while standing in line, before going to bed at night, after arising in the morning, or while simply relaxing in an easy chair with eyes closed.

When mental imagery buffs regularly pretend they are doing it right, away from the sites where the actual activity is practiced, they are capable of gaining accelerated improvement of their physical skills and personal body language. The payoff for the use of visualization is the obvious discovery of a lifetime learning process for gaining higher levels of performance in a very short period of time.

Now let's take a closer look at the "doing it right" pretend practice process and how to use it.

Imitating Success Sounds

Every physical movement has its own rhythmic success sounds. An expansion of creativity occurs as one organizes one's own vocal renditions of "doing it right" sounds. The sounds of a successful volleyball serve would be the toss, the jump, the pause and *pow!* A proper tennis ground stroke would be racquet back, racquet back, bounce, *pow!* A basketball free throw could sound like this: *Bounce-a-bounce-a-bounce* … *ahhhh* (deep breath) … *shoooooo* (ball in the air) … *swish* (ball going through the net).

Note: When holding a sheet of paper with one hand, slapping it with the other makes a sound identical to a ball passing through a net. This concept is a popular part of kid's play that can be observed when they ride imaginary horses (oftentimes while astride broomsticks) to the verbal sounds of *bogety ... bogety ... bogety* or *clipity-clop ... clipty-clop.*

A discussion on sounds of success would not be complete without a glance at the grandest of all my creative efforts—encouraging the use of mental imagery. Through the shared preparation of personalized self-motivation recordings, hundreds of students at UCSD and athletes in the greater community were able to experience accelerated improvement of their physical skills and mental attitudes.

A few years prior to joining the physical education department at UC San Diego, I was lured into the clutches of a pyramid scheme, and while attending a company motivation seminar, I purchased a motivation package with a thick manual and a dozen half-hour-long cassette tapes repeating (word for word) all the written information in the manual. The manufacturer of the tapes claimed that by listening to the recordings over and over again (they called it "forced repetition"), one would be motivated to achieve his or her predetermined goals. After a few weeks, rather than gaining heated motivation, I began questioning the effectiveness of repeatedly listening to the same information I had earlier read. I gave the tapes and manual away, but I kept the concept in the back of my mind.

In a few years, I came across the idea of using the forced repetition idea as a "sounds of success" technique for my mental imagery lessons. The recorded tape concept was a big hit with students. Most importantly, it gave me the opportunity to engage in a special, amazing, and innovative student–teacher association. The personalized recordings included favorite upbeat music, impromptu teacher and student remarks and readings, hearty group laffter, commitment to the use of enthusiasm gestures, and, lastly, twenty back-to-back voiced rhythms of perfect athletic movements. The following materials are needed to prepare this fantastic learning experience:

1. Two recording machines
2. One blank tape
3. At least two favorite songs per participant
4. A brief prepared paragraph of specific goal pursuits
5. Recorded sounds of hearty group laffter
6. Assorted sounds spelled on laffter flash cards
7. The individual movement success rhythms to be used

Here is the order of activities used to prepare personalized audio motivation success materials:

1. Seat participants so all are in range of the microphone.
2. Load recorders, one with a blank tape and the other with the facilitator's up-beat musical recording.
3. Begin recording with the facilitator's music playing in the background for fifteen seconds. Now lower the music volume so it can still be heard, while the facilitator then makes a brief impromptu statement like "Hi, Bruce, I'm so happy to assist in preparing this motivation experience for you." Then continue with remaining remarks, and end with "Replay these sounds to overcome moments of doubt and frustration, to reinforce your positive spirit, and most importantly to pretend practice using sounds of your athletic success." Now turn up the volume for another fifteen seconds.
4. At this point, place the participant's music in the appropriate recording machine and play the tune for fifteen seconds, and then lower the volume as before. The participant then says, "You know, Hubba, you are right; I am very wise, gifted, and confident and will achieve all my future goals!" Then continue with remaining remarks, and end with "I will utilize this recording to pick me up when I need a boost, celebrate the high moments I experience,

and pretend practice the skills I desire to perfect!" And again, turn the music up for another fifteen seconds.

5. Now repeat item number 4 by placing the facilitator's second song in the recorder. Play the music for another fifteen seconds, and then lower the volume once more, while the facilitator reads a favorite poem or positive comment, ending with the music returning to its original volume

6. Repeat activity number five, but this time using the participant's second tape while the participant reads his or her favorite poem;

7. Next, replace the music tape with the group laffter tape and play it in the background as participants join in celebrating during three to five minutes of continuous sounds of wild and exciting laffter. A selected participant prompts the group's laffter by flashing laffter flash cards to coordinate the sounds of extreme joy.

8. The final recorded activity is, of course, the participant's own voiced series of twenty back-to-back sounds of the success they desire to achieve.

This sequence of mental imagery involvement is a most interesting, awesome, and positive exercise promoting creative and effective student–teacher relations. Amend the process to suit your individual needs, and see how it will work for you; it sure worked wonders for me!

Video Replay

Video replay and photography have long been methods of providing feedback on "doing it right" movements. However, these techniques can be expensive and are unable to provide feedback on an immediate basis. Audio recordings are useful when sounds of success are recorded and imitated for twenty back-to-back repetitions. These sounds can be listened to with eyes closed while relaxing in a favorite reclining chair, while standing in a long line at the market, or while alone in the empty area where the real-life physical actions will take place.

Mirror Drills

Viewing "doing it right" movements in front of mirrors is cost effective and provides immediate feedback of imagined feats. Even greater use of this concept is to view "doing it right" images while performing in front of mirror or window reflections in the patio or at the mall. While teaching tennis, softball, and officiating classes at UCSD, I designed a four-sided mirror box used as a station to allow students to observe images of themselves performing their body mechanics in correct fashion.

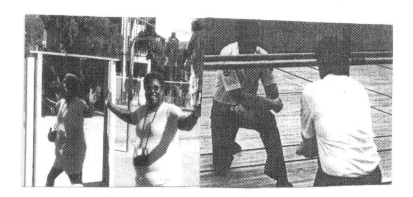

When I found many students were reluctant to move in front of the mirrors, I was able to ease their hesitations by teaming with them while we shared hearty side-by-side laffs in the mirror box. After two or three class meetings of hearty laff drills, students were able to more comfortably pretend practice in the mirror machine.

The Mind's TV Screen

Early introduction of visualization techniques to my beginning tennis classes found me instructing students to go home, assume a relaxed position, and try to view themselves doing tennis moves correctly on a wall in their home. Believe it or not, one graduate student majoring in psychology, who had been unable to master any of the basic tennis strokes after weeks of instruction, was able to actually see herself performing successful tennis strokes on her walls at home. A few days later, as I worked with her on stroke drills, assuming she would continue to perform poorly, I was shocked to no end as she hit a smashing forehand, with more speed than I could have ever imagined, directly at the net top and toward my groin area. Class members participating in the drill were amazed at what they saw, and even more so at the animated gestures I displayed attempting to dodge the ball's flight. Fortunately, the tennis ball slammed into the net, and injury to my body parts was avoided! After the laffing at Hubba was over, she explained to the class how she felt her "mind's eye" wall practice was the cause for her awesome accelerated stroke improvement.

Over the years, I have noticed that encouraging others to explore pretend practice exercises has oftentimes been an extremely difficult task. But most recently, I have experienced two rewarding visualization instances. Coincidentally, I have had recent chats with two former students who bragged to me about the marvelous thrills they receive by encouraging their children to successfully utilize the same pretend practice lessons I shared with them. Now how's that for deep and heavy student–teacher feedback?

Non-sport-related pretend practice drills can aid in the accelerated mastery of other physical skills and personal attitudes, including keyboarding, musical talents, positive gesturing, and self-esteem, just to name a few. Mirror imagery exercises can enhance the quality of one's laffter sounds and facial expressions. A full-sized copy of a keyboard can be placed on a table and used for imagination practice to improve the speed and accuracy of ones' keyboarding skills. What do you desire others to see when you interact with them? By regularly acting out the positive images and attitudes (body language) you want to share with others, you expose yourself to the lifetime ability to accelerate the learning of the actions and mannerisms you desire to master!

Chapter 7

Reflections of an Enthusiasm Mentor

The primary expectation in previous chapters has been to discuss ideas capable of empowering folks to experience greater feelings of human success, personal enthusiasm, and joy galore. This chapter offers reflections on the decades of pioneer concepts, reeducation, and success experiences that made me who I am today. At the conclusion of each reflection, space is available for readers to write in their own reflections on the reflections.

Reflection 1

Do you have a purpose in life for which you are intended?
Once you have established a purpose in life for yourself, you have taken a major step toward enriching your self-motivation to achieve your planned goals. So don't delay; organize your personal goal-setting plans today. Simply speaking, put your mind on notice for the future desires related to your family, career, housing, education, leisure time, and retirement conditions. Too many people are content to merely leave their life choices to chance. But those who cement their thoughts into a plan of action are able to gain the "gonnas" which in time mature to the "I did its." These efforts allow users to become more creative by equipping them with the ability to more routinely change their thoughts into things!

So often we delay making our life goal planning decisions until tomorrow or until bad times get better. But often that tomorrow never comes and the tough times drag on and on.

There is never a need to put your future career options on the back burner. Everyone should focus on their family, workplace character, future living conditions, and retirement lifestyle. While pursuing current obligations, never get caught without a definite predetermined plan of action for the future. If you don't have major goals to pursue and commit yourself to, select any you would follow if you did know. Establish directions, even if you may want to change them in the future. Nothing is wrong with updating your directions somewhere down the road, and if you do so, you will have activated your goal-striving mechanism, ensuring future goal pursuits will advance in an easier manner. Surely times and conditions will change, but always keep in mind that a ship carrying valuable cargo will never sail from port without a final destination in mind.

<u>Personally Speaking</u>

My educational experiences never provided me with the knowledge of goal-setting strategies and how they influence later life conditions. By either luck or chance, my life successes thus far have just happened to fall into place. It wasn't until I reached preretirement age that I really began to think about my future life conditions. I am thankful I was able to receive a more-than-adequate pension and health benefits from a very adequate package provided from my employer (UC San Diego). So many people are unable to enjoy such a favored advantage. Thanks to previous "luck," my wife, Edna, and I are enjoying a quality of retired life far beyond any we anticipated during our earlier years. We have relocated from San Diego to Arkansas, where living is easy, catfish are biting, gas is cheap, and traffic is oh so slow! For those of you still in the early stages of planning your future life plans, take heed and be sure you make it a priority to seriously prepare for your "sunset years."

Brief Reflections on the Reflection: _____

_____

_____

_____

_____

Reflection 2

What are your fondest passions?

We should identify and give special attention to the positive passions in our lives. The things you enjoy the most and bring you the greatest satisfaction should become the centerpieces of your lifelong ambitions. Somewhere in your hobbies, career, and leisure activities lies the foundation for your passion pursuits. Be careful when organizing these endeavors, and make sure to include only things dear to you. Avoid decisions following the whims of others, including family, friends, and associates. Satisfying the expectations of others should never be the prime factor in selecting your self-fulfilling options. Just think of all the persons who never fully actualized themselves because they chased passions urged or arranged by others. An added thought is to search out the possibilities of involving your greatest passions into business ventures for financial gain.

Personally Speaking

Over the younger years of my adult life, I saw no need to organize my life passions. While supporting my family was my major concern, I became very excited about the sports officiating class I was teaching at UC San Diego. It turned out that the success of a class training students to become dynamic sports officials created an innovative and exciting career passion and timely vehicle benefiting me and my family. Prior to joining the physical education department at UC San Diego, I was able to gain three years of summer employment as a professional Minor League Baseball umpire. The travel involved during three summers (1969 to 1971) enabled my family and me (traveling in our Aljo trailer) to vacation in a half dozen western states. Three years later, I had the opportunity to serve as an umpire in the Alaska Baseball League during the summer months of 1974 to 1976. Each season, my family would join me for two weeks, to once again vacation in a most interesting area of the USA. The impact of these summer adventures was immeasurable for my children. From the Snake River (Idaho); to Yellowstone Park (Wyoming); to Denali Park (Alaska); to Reno, Nevada; to the farmlands of the San Joaquin Valley (Bakersfield to Lodi, California), we enjoyed a span of rare family summer fun experienced by few families. Years later, my wife and I had heartwarming experiences while watching television when our children (then in their teens) would shout, "Hey Mom and Dad, that's where we were!"

Brief Reflections on the Reflection: _____

_____

_____

_____

_____

Reflection 3

Do you please others before you please yourself?

How do you answer this question? In my mind, too many persons are obsessed with pleasing others before tending to themselves. It is important for us to consider putting our own well-being first, and that of others next. To be a good "people person" is the popular ambition for most persons, and rightfully so. Have you ever been waiting in line at the market and had a person behind you clip your heels with his or her shopping cart? Did you make that person aware of this annoying gesture, or did you remain silent in order to not upset them? If we assert our personal feelings to others in a kindly manner, we increase our self-confidence and conversation skills with others. Some may look at this as "ego-tripping" of sorts, but I see it as a kind of positive ego-tripping. Such expressions create an enhanced quality of positive behavior while respecting the feelings of others. Yes, I am a positive supporter for the idea that you should consider yourself first and display quality people-person skills at the same time. As one designs creative ways to activate positive ego-tripping skills, he or she proceeds to become a more dynamic influence within his or her circle of influences.

<u>Personally Speaking</u>

I have always considered myself a strong "people person." My desire to promote joy and enthusiasm has made it easy for me to reach out to others and draw their attention to the ideas I share. Early in my professional career, as I became better acquainted with strategies leading to personal success, I learned to make sure I placed myself first (in regard to fulfilling my own personal goals), and in so doing, I enhanced my efforts to mentor and share enthusiasm and hearty laffter with others. Another word of advice to those who would like to progress their "self-first" talents is to avoid making important decisions solely on the opinions of others. Of course it is wise to solicit thoughts from time to time, but only as recommendations, not for immediate actions. Many of my creative actions have been rather controversial, and were often challenged by those I approached for counsel. While I appreciated receiving their thoughts, after reviewing them, I most often opted for my gut-felt courses of action. As I look back, I see that the results of my gut actions have worked out very well; and on each occasion, these actions reinforced the idea of positive ego-tripping!

Brief Reflections on the Reflection: _____
_____
_____
_____
_____

Reflection 4

Can you turn setbacks into stepping stones?

We all encounter setbacks and frustrations as we pursue our daily endeavors. How many times have you fallen victim to stinging heartbreaks, hardships, and other negative experiences? How did you react to these situations? How long does it take you to regain your positive thoughts after a mind-boggling event? Depending on the individual, the time it takes to recover emotionally from a major setback may be a few hours, a day or two, or even several weeks. While unfortunate twists in our lives cannot be avoided, they can be less painful if we train ourselves to turn negatives into positives by mastering "remember 2B positive" techniques. The benefits of reversing negatives and turning them into positives have been cited in earlier chapters. Turning negatives into positives helps people deal with the disappointing experiences they may have from time to time. In order to gain mastery of positive life skill habits, it is important to explore ways to turn your setbacks into positive experiences.

<u>Personally Speaking</u>

This reach toward eternal enthusiasm greatly enhanced my ability to teach and mentor enthusiasm and laffter-connection concepts. These techniques evolved in spite of my losing four career positions as a result of the inability of others to understand the nature of my enthusiastic behaviors. I trained myself to maintain upbeat attitudes amid adverse and trying conditions. In spite of the negative feedback from others, I developed what I refer to as positive ego-tripping as a survival technique. After recovering from the second setback, I began to realize that no matter how bad things may seem at the moment, they will eventually get better. In each situation, I found myself rebounding to a place far better than where I had been before. In later situations, I found it less stressful and easier to survive periods between darkness and sunshine, while exploring new options for the future. In order to be better prepared to maintain your sanity and self-control during difficult periods, consider developing personal methods for turning your setbacks into stepping stones.

Brief Reflections on the Reflection: _____

_____

_____

_____

_____

Reflection 5

Does anyone ever win a spraying fight with a skunk?

Have you ever been sprayed by a skunk? Can you imagine what a low-down and mind-boggling experience this would be? However, day in and day out, so many people attempt to win spraying fights with the skunks in their life. It is important to stand up for the things we believe in; but on the other hand, before rushing into emotionally charged actions, defending our beliefs, we must make sure to wage our battles wisely. Most often, misunderstandings with skunks include conflicts with the authority figures we face every day, including our parents, our friends, our teachers, our coaches, the police, our coworkers, and our supervisors, to name a few. Every now and then, most often by chance, a person may win a spraying fight with a skunk, but most often skunks will rule.

Let's glance at a few situations where the authority figures are almost certain to win. (Note: The reference to skunks is no way related to authority figures actually being skunks. It is just a saying identifying the odds of losing confrontations with various authoritative resources).

1. Parents denying their child's desire to go steady
2. Heated discussions with others who take positions opposite to yours in such areas as race, politics, religion, war or peace, and gender issues

3. Arguing vigorously against police instructions
4. Initiating strong verbal communication with persons known for resorting to violent activities

To prevent skunks from spraying, remember to remain cool, calm, and collected and place your emotions on hold for later review.

Personally Speaking

As I look back on my past, I see that too many times I failed to heed the wisdom in this reflection. So often, out of pride, stubbornness, or outright anger, I waged senseless battles with a countless number of skunks; and I never triumphed a single time! Several of these conflicts led to the loss of employment positions. Fortunately for me (but not necessarily so for many I have known), I was able to bounce back after the wounds from my skunk fights healed. I cannot guarantee similar silver linings will align themselves for you as they did for me. In the future, take the time to carefully evaluate the need to wage forces against the skunk populations in your life. Will the cost of losing a skunk brawl be more than you are willing to pay? Are you properly equipped with the resources to regain any losses you might incur?

Finally, mention must be given to the various tensions arising between significant others from time to time. Like myself, my spouse is a very strong-minded individual and is never hesitant to voice her opinions on any "hot topics" occurring in our home. About forty years ago, I discovered the reality that a man seldom, if ever, wins a disagreement with his woman. (Let it be known that I am not implying my wife is a skunk.) Keeping this in mind has greatly reduced the number of misunderstandings we could have had over the past two decades of our fifty-three years of matrimony. This philosophy also aided me some twenty years ago when I returned to the classroom as an elementary school teacher. Over the next seven years, I was under the direction of three women principals who, like my wife, had solid-minded tendencies. I immediately recognized how fortunate I was to have an awareness of how to work in harmony with them, because of the strategies I was using at home! However, just to keep an allegiance to my male ego, about every tenth time my wife and I have conflicting views, I will take a stand, just to satisfy my male instincts. I must utter my thanks to Anthony Maslow and Carl Rogers for the wisdom of their approaches to humanistic psychology, which I was exposed to during my graduate studies for a master's degree in counselor education back in 1975.

Forever remember that the odds of claiming victory in spraying fights with skunks are poor!

Brief Reflections on the Reflection: _____

_____

_____

_____

_____

Reflection 6

Would you dare to laff ten seconds longer every day?

I cannot imagine anyone reading chapter 2 and not leaving with an understanding of how hearty laffter can enhance the quality of his or her daily life. If you buy into the fact that laffter has the ability to heal, reduce anger, ease stress, and inspire positive outlooks, it is time for you to increase the volume and frequency of your laffter. There's nothing left for you to do but *do it!* Eagerly bring more joy and happiness to the world by discovering your favorite laffing face (you can find it in front of the favorite mirror of your life), and then begin sharing it ten seconds longer every day.

Personally Speaking

I have to confess that my many years of spreading joy and enthusiasm have offered me many heartwarming and enjoyable experiences. It has made no difference who the audiences have been: kindergarten classes, sports teams, senior citizens, bank employees, professionals, or community members. The results have always been the same: loads of shared enthusiasm and laffter. I have had opportunities to share my hearty laffter in many communities, in many states, and on several West Indies islands. Sharing my jovial and infectious laffter has been very self-satisfying, and I marvel at the positive impact I have on the lives of others as they laff, sing, and perform gestures of extreme enthusiasm. Perhaps the most rewarding thing I observe is the looks on the faces of folks as they display amazing images of hearty laffter while swallowing large doses of Hubba Jubba joy and enthusiasm. Listed below are evaluative remarks made by students in several personal health and safety classes I taught at the University of Arkansas–Pine Bluff a few years ago. The early chapters of the class textbook covered a range of topics similar to those we have discussed in earlier chapters.

I learned about the importance of enthusiasm and how laughter can make me feel better.

In this class, I have learned that laughter can be used to better my life anywhere and at any time I choose to use it.

I have learned laughter opens the door for making new relationships. I plan to use laughter to make life better for myself and others.

I have never laughed more than I have in this class. Laughing more has made me a better person and now helps me get through the bad days I run into.

Hubba has everyone in the class laughing every day. I knew laughter could reduce stress, so now, whenever I am stressed out, I "laff it up."

I learned that laughter is more powerful than I thought. I now use it to make me feel better when I'm having a bad day.

I have learned how important laughter is in the makeup of a happy day. Laughter is a medicine I can use to stay positive regardless of the circumstances.

I now use laughter more frequently. I want to live a long and happy life, so I laugh at myself more, make light of things I have no control over, view the world differently, and always remember to "laff it up."

Several of the important things I have learned about are the characteristics of a good laugh, that gelotology is the study of laughter, and that wide-open-mouth laughs are the best of all.

I have made a conscious effort to laugh more, and it has really made my life go a lot smoother.

Hubba always came to class humming a happy tune; provided interesting stories, lectures, and discussions; and made us sing happy songs and make happy stickers and draw laughing faces on paper plates.

I've learned that laughing eases stress and tension and can help me remember to be positive, and that whenever my day needs a lift, I need to "laff it up!"

Brief Reflections on the Reflection: _____

_____
_____
_____
_____

Reflection 7

Can you afford quality pretend practice time?

While the values of pretend practice have been reviewed earlier, here are a few more thoughts on this dynamic mental process. Most persons I introduce to the idea of mental imagery agree it sounds interesting, but due to circumstances I have yet to figure out, it is difficult getting them involved in serious pretend practice activities. On the other hand, those who do commit themselves to acts of pretend practice are able to experience accelerated achievement of the skills they desire to actualize.

Visualization concepts are nothing new and have been passed down over the ages to our current generations. Asian cultures have imagined hands traveling through bricks. Africans imitate lifelike images and movements of the animal life in their regions through their dance and rituals. In the West Indies culture, their voodoo practices use keen imagination to heal and influence their people—not to inflict harm upon others, as media resources often portray.

Mental rehearsal drills have the ability to improve the development of our physical skills and personal attitudes in an accelerated fashion. From an enthusiasm-building perspective, imagination drills not only promote rapid results but also boost feelings of self-confidence that lead to higher levels of enthusiasm development. The range of visualization opportunities is huge and is limited only by the creativity and motivation of its users. Are you ready to explore efforts to strengthen your skills and attitudes through the use of pretend practice exercises? If so, begin to further research information on visualization topics and allow yourself to explore one of the greatest life skills tools in the world today. Commit yourself to the use of pretend practice exercises for furthering your personal development, and you will find yourself becoming more and more successful at everything you do!

Personally Speaking

The most important factor in designing my enthusiasm-building philosophy started while I was using mental imagery techniques in the physical education classes I was teaching at UC San Diego. Thanks to the rapid student success and the presence of my bigger-than-life example of enthusiasm in action, mutual admiration relationships developed between my students and me. As things turned out, most students readily accepted the invitation to utilize mental imagery drills to enhance the quality of their tennis serves, softball throws, umpiring "out" calls, varsity sport skills and overall positive attitudes. The ideas of bioreflective feedback (mirror box drills), audio-tonal rhythms (recorded sounds of skill success), and hand-crafted mementos ("remember 2B positive" collages and motivation tapes) combine to create amazing accelerated success endeavors. Add to these ingredients the dynamic and enthusiastic Hubba Jubba spirit, and quickened improvement of motor skills and self-confidence are guaranteed. The cost to enjoy the fruits of mental imagery use cannot be beaten; anyone can afford it, because the cost is free. You can't afford not to miss this treat!

Brief Reflections on the Reflection: _____

_____

_____

_____

_____

Reflection 8

Do you burn bridges behind you?
Have you ever made hasty decisions and later realized things may have been better if an alternate choice had been selected? It is a common impulse for people to make flash decisions, especially when under the influence of stress or anger. I have been in such situations several times, and in hindsight I see that maybe it would

have been better for me to step back, take a brief breath, and hold off on making those speedy decisions. I now believe it is wiser to take time out to evaluate existing circumstances before rushing into actions that may not be best for you in the long run. Another thing to consider is teaching yourself to admit the mistakes you make, recognize them, correct them, and let go of any allegiances to them in the future. Ignoring our errors and refusing to admit them causes many folks to get stuck in a rut and face more negative outcomes than they should. The ability to own up to mistakes and move on is not a symbol of weakness, as many claim. More positive responses to our misfortunes and disagreements allow us to avoid the consequences of burning bridges behind us.

You may want to seek the opinions of wise people you know. You may also want to use those people as sounding boards for alternatives rather than making hasty decisions. Always be sure the final actions you pursue are your own and are not solely based upon the thoughts you receive from others. The moral of this reflection is to refrain from making immediate emotional decisions in critical situations. Take time out to consider the results of the difficult decisions you make, and welcome advice from selected trusted persons.

Personally Speaking

It was earlier mentioned I have survived several situations where I burned bridges behind me. My fleet resignations from several career positions were made on an "I'll show them" basis, and there I was, unemployed and wondering what I would do next. Fortunately, these incidents turned out well for me, but I had no influence on these lucky results. While I cherish the lucky breaks I experienced, I now understand luck is for chumps. And oh, what a chump I was. Today I am careful to make life-impacting decisions with more patience and concern for how they will influence my future. My list of trusted persons is very short, and most often I rely on input from the wife of my life when vital decisions must be made. Although we often have to compromise our ideas in the end, it is only fair, because most of these outcomes will affect us both!

Brief Reflections on the Reflection: _____

_____

_____

_____

_____

Reflection 9

What do you know about what you eat?

There is an ageless saying that goes something like this: "We are what we eat." Are you in the habit of monitoring the food you eat? Do you read the labels when purchasing items at the grocery store? A positive change in our time finds many people becoming more aware of the food they put in their mouths. However, most people still fail to make this vital health choice. It must be noted that diets of certain ethnic groups and those with extreme lifestyles are more likely to exhibit certain health conditions. Heart disease, diabetes, obesity, and a wide range of other related illnesses exist as a result of the worldwide lack of proper eating habits. To live a longer and healthier life, it is important to know the values of the foods we eat. If you have yet to do so, begin to examine the amount of fat, sodium, cholesterol, carbohydrates, and calories you consume each day. Contact your medical doctor for further suggestions on how to pursue a healthier lifestyle. The knowledge of the food passing through your mouth each day can add years and zest to your life. Forever remember: "We are what we eat!"

Personally Speaking

Make no mistake about it; I am a living example of how diet neglect can cause major health problems. I have always exhibited (and still do) a body profile of enthusiastic girth. (What a creative way to say I have always been overweight.) It wasn't until the turn of the century, when my body became affected by type 2 diabetes, that I began monitoring the foods I placed in my mouth. My doctor informed me that if I lost weight and minimized my carbohydrate intake, there was a good chance he would not have to put me on any diabetes medicines. Nine years later, after shedding close to 105 pounds (I should still lose 50 more), my blood sugar, cholesterol, blood pressure, and heart rate are back in a normal range.

After moving from California to Arkansas in 2006, I faced another health crisis. I ignored visiting a new doctor in Arkansas for more than a year. After my wife's urging to see a doctor, I finally visited one, only to discover my blood pressure was a staggering 200/112. This was definitely a major health hazard, because a normal blood pleasure reading is 130/60. This situation evolved over a period of time as I cut my carbohydrate count and freely consumed lower-carb items, including processed meats galore. Little did I know the deli meats, bacon, and sausages I was eating were laced with sodium, which sent my blood pressure off the charts. All is well now, as my blood pressure and blood sugar levels have returned to a normal level. Do you know what your blood pressure is? To be safe, you should check your blood pressure at least two times a month. Over the past several months, my diet awareness has enabled me to lose more than thirty-five pounds, and I have pledged to maintain my successful diet habits as well as double my weekly exercise time. At over seventy-six years of age, I am a giant, economy-size image of how important it is to be aware of the foods entering your stomach. I enthusiastically urge you to monitor the foods entering your stomach, too!

Brief Reflections on the Reflection: _____

_____

_____

_____

_____

Chapter 8

Applying Enthusiasm Concepts

This concluding chapter reviews options for advancing your initial enthusiasm/laffter concepts to a higher level. While some items have been previously discussed, let's review a few items on how to maintain and implement progressive life skill habits.

Desire to learn and develop lifetime talents and skills.

Personal growth should be a major part of every person's success philosophy. Lifetime learning enables one to maintain and enhance the quality of his or her career endeavors, personal attitudes, and communication abilities. Providing continued enthusiasm growth includes upgrading knowledge and techniques as a stepping stone toward higher levels of life skills mastery. Throughout the ages, great philosophers and leadership gurus have constantly promoted the wisdom of pursuing continued learning. Also associated with lifelong learning is the actualization of self-esteem. The more knowledge you gain, the more esteemed you become. Moreover, your sense of creativity is equally expanded, providing you with a greater ability to design and implement progressive actions for yourself and others. Always remember this piece of Hubba Jubba advice: "Creativity is me and you too!"

Never fret or give up when the going gets tough; and it will.

One of the most frustrating things in life is to be stuck in the clutches of lengthy and unenjoyable career or personal situations.

Design your ultimate career goals and personal dreams for the purpose of gaining peace of mind and joy galore. Always keep in mind that other people and unexpected events will cross your paths, causing you to possibly lose focus of your desired ambitions. But fret not; keep your "dream shoes" on, and stay true to what you believe in becoming. Moreover, occasions may arise where you find yourself amid employment and social conditions far from your ideal plans. In such instances, you must view these circumstances as temporary stepping stones toward your fond and more rewarding future goals. In order to stay on track and survive negative influences, equip yourself with a gamut of enthusiasm and laffter mementos reminding you 2B positive, and in due time you will reconnect with your roadway to success!

The combination of spiritual resources, self-determination, and motivational mementos forms a can't-miss guidance system directing you to the mountaintops you dare to climb. Use these things to keep yourself from falling victim to frustrations and despair. The key to continued treks to the high peaks you desire to conquer is never forgetting the deep and foggy valleys from which you have climbed. A vivid example of this concept is found in a poem by Langston Hughes entitled "Mother to Son." Make a copy of the poem to place in your backpack, wallet, or purse to refer to as an added motivation resource amid the setbacks and heartaches you will face along the way to your stars!

Create a schedule for all daily activities.

While good ideas are important, they are nothing until put into action. Too often grand ideas go down the drain because their originator neglected to see them to their end. Time management is essential for achieving human success. In today's hustle and bustle times, it is easy to become distracted and lose sight of your visions. To lessen the occurrences of goal distractions, it is important to maintain a strong grip on time management techniques. Those with modern technology skills need only keep daily schedules on their cell phone or computer. Commit yourself to the possession of a personal date book, calendar, or electronic device noting your daily activities, along with their scheduled times and places. Place your schedule next to your bed at the end of the day. Prior to falling asleep and upon waking in the morning, review your obligations for the day. In cases where scheduled events are cancelled, immediately enter the new day, time, and place of the rescheduled date. Also be sure to check your personal schedule several times each day, to make sure you are on track with planned activities. A well-planned daily schedule includes such entries as

- morning wake-up time
- meal and snack times
- selected break times
- time allowed for transportation needs
- items to complete during the day
- time blocks for classes and study time
- job assignments
- personal business
- relaxation time
- social activities

Include time for visualization exercises each day.

As mentioned before, creative visualization has been very, very good to me! I urge you to make the process work for you too. Research shows the human brain is used only to a minimum of its full potential. One sure way to expand the use of your brain's function is to regularly use visualization exercises. Over the years, I have discovered oftentimes it's difficult to engage persons in the exploration of new ideas. Outside of the instruction I provide under classroom conditions, it has often been a struggle to engage folks with pretend practice drills. However, those who explore pretend practice activities experience the exciting ability to accelerate the learning and improvement of their physical and personal attitude skills. In keeping with the upgrading of post-enthusiasm skills, successful use of visualization techniques takes its users to a higher level when they begin to share their newfound knowledge with others.

Share your developing skills with others.

Here comes the recurring theme of sharing with others again. What good is it to have guidelines for achieving human success in the palm of your hand and not pass them on to those around you? If a major need for the world is to discover and develop more persons able to promote the enthusiasm–laffter connection, then the next greatest thing is to ensure they thrive on cloning their motivation talents in the lives of others. The power of an enthusiasm sharer is not only in the ability to inspire others, but in the ability to teach them how to inspire others too!

Organize gatherings of others interested in sharing enthusiasm.

Consider meeting with others eager to improve their motivation skills too. If two heads are better than one, then it goes without saying three heads are better than two. Therefore, developing enthusiasm "think tank" activities is a unique way to broaden the appreciation of enthusiasm and laffter concepts. The creation of such groups with enthusiasm-sharing on their minds allows for regular gatherings to discuss and develop ways to promote greater gestures of joy and positive attitudes. Weekly or monthly meetings (depending on the group's enthusiasm for enthusiasm) provide opportunities to share the recent experiences group members have encountered.

Sessions should focus on specific observations and personal reactions related to recent episodes they have experienced, and their plans for the same in the future. Since joint visits with enthusiasm mentors may result in lengthy rant-and-rave sessions, following is a suggested agenda for gatherings of enthusiasm mentors:

1. Informal social mixer time and dynamic opening activity
2. Creative introductions by all attending

3. Setting of a time limit to review recent participant experiences
4. Questions and responses to review items
5. Brainstorm session on thoughts for future actions
6. Closing dynamic team-building activity

An extended option for the group is to create joint gatherings for those they mentor. What can be more exciting than providing learning and social experiences featuring enthusiasm mentors in joint activities with those they influence?

Achieve a new skill, then another, then another, then another.

This application is extremely important in sustaining lasting achievements of human success. Once one acquires the knowledge and applications for becoming successful, one has the ability to transfer his or her formula to other lifestyle conditions. To become an active enthusiasm mentor and then slack off is a violation of the concept's code. Understanding even a single key to success equips one with the power to invent one success saga after another. History teaches us that past success heroes have lost their initial fruits of success, only to, in due time, regain their lost levels of success. Therefore, to discover ways to inspire and mentor enthusiasm for others is to possess a ticket to pursue unlimited success skills and talents. A philosophy for achieving the status of eternal enthusiasm equips one with the credentials to translate it to any number of their future success aspirations.

Never be satisfied with average human success.

Today graveyards hold the remains of so many persons who could have achieved so much more if they had only possessed a passion for becoming the best they could be. Everyone is born a star, but unfortunately many people lack the confidence to tell themselves so! The combination of goal-setting, enthusiasm, creativity, and self-esteem (of course the most important of these is enthusiasm; it's the all in all) is powerful for maximizing one's human potential and happiness. So why is the road toward maximum human success so often ignored? Do any of these following reasons relate to you?

1. Lack of knowledge on how to achieve human success
2. Satisfaction in being just like others
3. Fear of standing out from the crowd
4. Comfort in being modest and shy rather than outgoing and energetic
5. Fear of making mistakes and enduring related embarrassments
6. General laziness and lack of motivation to be a leader or achiever
7. Peer encouragement to avoid personal growth activities
8. Tendency to procrastinate
9. Failure to recognize the worthwhile value of becoming the best
10. Absence of association with positive role models, peers or friends

To the enthusiasm mentor, the opportunity to reverse the attitudes listed above is the purpose for which they are intended. There is no greater feeling of personal achievement and happiness than a mentor of enthusiasm viewing the first signs of self-confidence and positive esteem beginning to grow in the minds and actions of those they influence.

Fear not competition; it encourages greater success and joy.

How many times have you heard someone say, "Winning is not important, but how you play the game is?" Assuming this is true, it is reasonable to assume that if you play the game of life with enthusiasm, you can't lose. A popular thought in the minds of many views the desire to win as a negative condition. How do you feel about advocating noncompetitive practices; is competition good or bad? Oftentimes, a noncompetitive attitude weakens the desire in those who strive to become their best. The passion for exploring far reaches of human potential is a healthy experience if it is pursued to gain higher personal goals. When goal pursuits create friction and controversy for others, they are not of a positive nature. The ability to face healthy competition is a reality for those desiring to achieve better family, employment, and lifetime opportunities. Worthy competition is easy to explore when quality future achievements are well designed and frequently visualized, assisted by the display of numerous positive mementos and the ingestion of large doses of enthuuuuuuusiasm.

Career advancement comes easier to folks with multiple skills.

In keeping with the previous discussion of career endeavors, let us look at the value of establishing and maintaining sound workplace skills and habits. While some people despise assuming leadership responsibilities, others bask in chances to gain upward career mobility leading to supervisory positions. What are your thoughts on this occupational situation? Any of the following actions will equip one with the tools to establish the competitive edge in the race for career promotions and upward mobility:

1. Having a bad day? Then fake it to make it; no one needs to know.
2. Regularly come early and stay late.
3. Avoid work-site conflicts and gossip.
4. Complete courses and workshops to gain additional job-related skills.
5. Participate in all available in-service activities.
6. Attend one professional meeting a year (even at your expense, if necessary).
7. Volunteer to present sessions and hold offices with professional organizations in your field.
8. Promote work-site special-interest lunchtime (brown bag) or after-work activities.
9. Schedule regular rap sessions with friends possessing positive work ethics.

10. Share joy and enthusiasm throughout your workplace every day!

Enjoy what you do; it nurtures greater wellness.

There is nothing more exciting, rewarding, and stress-free than enjoying what you do from day to day. Those fortunate enough to have enjoyable employment options, positive relationships, and solid self-esteem are able to experience worthy living conditions for themselves and their families. Because of recent hardships including armed conflicts abroad, economic despair, job layoffs, a career crisis, and inadequate health care conditions, options for personal enjoyment have become increasingly difficult for large numbers of people. The sadness in today's madness is the varied uncertainties impeding achievement efforts for those who are ready to activate enhanced enthusiasm skills. While willpower, spiritual zest, and enthusiasm mementos have great merit, they are less applicable when folks are dealing with unemployment, strained budgets, lackluster benefits, and family members in harm's way.

However, the concept of sharing enthusiasm and laffter is a powerful asset for those daring to embrace it in spite of the difficulties they must also overcome. What is the condition of your life's story? How important is enthusiasm enrichment to you? Are you able to dedicate yourself to becoming an enthusiasm mentor today?

Just Have Fun!

Isn't fun what life is all about anyway? When we are having fun at home, work, play, or spiritual sites, everything is bright and rosy. These are the moments in our lives when we are experiencing joy, self-pride, confidence, and enthusiasm galore. But when our happiness is dealt a severe blow and the good moments fade away, who knows how long it will be before the void of good feelings return.

Now that you have an understanding about the enthusiasm–laffter connection and its related techniques, you are equipped with tools to easily enhance the quality of your creative and positive attitude skills. Lastly, create and display any number of handmade "remember 2B positive" mementos for backup resources, to remind you to hold strong to the goals and attitudes you need to ensure daily and lifelong personal success and happiness.

Summary

The Enthusiasm–Laffter Connection serves as a guide for persons who desire to improve the quality of their personal life skills. For readers who would like to take the wisdom in these pages to even a higher level, they can use the book as a resource for developing personalized techniques to mentor joy and enthusiasm with the persons they influence.

Enthusiasm is an important human life skills characteristic. Enthusiasm is a learnable skill, but very few programs exist for the specific purpose of teaching how to do so. What our world needs now is to include enthusiasm instruction in curricula at all educational institutions and all levels of workplace training. In future years, the competition for employment, leadership roles, and other career opportunities will become more competitive, so more emphasis will be based upon the positive nature of a person's oral and physical interview styles.

Hearty laffter is the best enthusiasm; and its uses and benefits have been advanced over the past thirty years through the field of gelotology (the scientific study of laffter). Always remember that the anatomy of a hearty laff is a wide-open-mouthed gesture, never a smile or grin. Big laffs can ease pain, lessen stress, lift spirits, and in general cause good things to happen. Be sure to select six laffter facts and immediately add them to your personal expressions of joy!.

The connection between laffs and enthusiasm is based upon the fact that hearty laffter is the greatest gesture of human enthusiasm.

Like enthusiasm, creativity has been equally ignored as a valuable life skill. Human creativity can be taught and mentored too. We tap into the creativity resources within us when we broaden the scope and use of our imagination. Examples of creativity exercises are available through the preparation of a variety of images reflecting positive attitude concepts. The Moss-Cess Success Profile and The Moss-Cess Success Process, motivation mementos, slogans, and other artwork demonstrate innovative usage of creativity. Lacking the possession of expert drawing skills is no excuse for not creating personalized artwork. The technological resources of our day are capable of producing excellent visual images for anyone desiring to do so!

Let's review several previously discussed actions for widening the creativity within us.

1. Design and use improved gestures of enthusiasm.
2. Research and develop any number of favorite laff sounds and facial gestures.
3. Become an advocate for creating "remember 2B positive" handmade motivation mementos, including stickers, posters, collages, and bookmarks. These items provide environmental influences to assist in maintaining 24-7 positive attitude conditions.
4. Learn to master visualization (i.e., pretend practice) activities to accelerate the learning of physical skills and personal attitudes.
5. Be sure to add any number of the twelve S's into your daily routine.
6. Everyone is born to be a star. How sad it is to know that so many people never get to become the star they were meant to be. Just like a star, enthusiastic persons shine, spread warmth, lead the way, and radiate positive vibes to those who know them. If you aren't already feeling like a star, start acting like you're one right away! Be a star wannabe today, and then become one in the tomorrows to come!
7. Challenge your knowledge of this book's content by responding to the reader's quiz.
8. Utilize the page at the end of this book referring to the list of relevant resources.

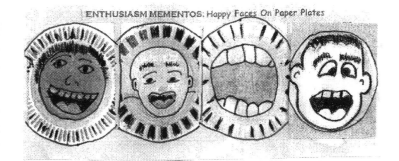

ENTHUSIASM MEMENTOS: Happy Faces On Paper Plates

Reader's Quiz

Challenge the learning you have gained by answering the quiz items below. The answers are available at the end of the quiz.

I. **True/False:** Circle *T* or *F* for each item.

1. T F Enthusiasm is a popular subject in school and workplace training programs.

2. T F Hubba Jubba learns as much from his students as they learn from him.

3. T F Two "remember 2B positive" items are stickers and happy paper plates.

4. T F It is impossible to teach a person to have better enthusiasm.

5. T F A major purpose in one's life is to have fun.

6. T F Most persons who have enthusiasm know how they got it.

7. T F A tip for gaining instant enthusiasm is to count backward from 100 to 1.

8. T F Hubba was a physical education teacher at UC San Diego.

9. T F The enthusiasm–laffter connection began in an officiating class.

10. T F Laffology is the scientific name for the study of laffter.

11. T F Hubba's officiating students at UC San Diego earned over $3 million.

12. T F Hearty laffter is the best enthusiasm.

13. T F If Coach says, "That's it," a mirror should be visited immediately.

14. T F Pretend practice works only during routine practice drills.

15. T F Today, Hubba shares his wisdom with the world.

II. **Fill-Ins:** Place the correct words in the blank spaces.

1. During a hearty laff, air passes over the vocal chords at ___ mph.

2. When repeated three times, the most used sound of laffter is ___ ___ ___.

3. Three other laff sounds are ___ ___ ___, ___ ___ ___, ___ ___ ___.

4. Hearty laffter is the greatest gesture of _____.

5. List two things laffter can do for you: _____, _____.

6. Name three "remember 2B positive" mementos: _____, _____, _____.

7. Deck your _____ and _____ with positive images.

8. Creativity is me and _____.

9. Hubba's success profile includes an Afro _____.

10. The words "I don't need you anymore" appear on the _____ _____.

11. Teachers use their supply stores to purchase what motivation items? _____.

12. The father of healing laffter was _____.

13. Hubba prints his stickers on _____ paper.

14. Hubba's student umps were summer interns in _____.

15. Today Hubba has expanded his classroom to the _____.

III.   **Matching:** Place the proper letters in spaces on the left.

1. __ Another name for visualization   A) *Pow*
2. __ In the beginning one must fake it   B) Sharing enthusiasm
3. __ What this book is all about   C) Psychology
4. __ One dozen enthusiasm techniques   D) *Swish*
5. __ Nonsport use of visualization   E) To make it
6. __ The crown jewel of our minds   F) Keyboard practice
7. __ The greatest *S* of all   G) Creativity
8. __ Watch "doing it right" practice   H) The twelve S's
9. __ Verbal sounds for riding a horse   I) Mirror drills
10. __ Verbal sound for successful free   J) I-2-I contact
    throws
11. __ Major of hard-hitting tennis   K) Label paper
    student
12. __ Hearty laffter is never a grin or a   L) Pretend practice
13. __ Motivation stickers are printed on   M) *Boogaty-boogaty*
14. __ Verbal sound for tennis success   N) Smile
15. __ One of the tips for instant   O) Sharing
    enthusiasm

IV.   **What I Will Do:** Five ways I will improve the quality of my laffter:

1. _____
2. _____
3. _____
4. _____
5. _____

V. **Happy Faces:** In the faces below, draw the correct mouths.

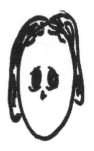 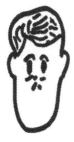 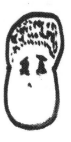 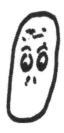

FROWN   SMILE   GRIN   HEARTY LAFF

Quiz Answers

True/False	Matching
1. F	1. L
2. T	2. E
3. T	3. B
4. F	4. H
5. T	5. F
6. F	6. G
7. F	7. O
8. T	8. I
9. T	9. M
10. F	10. D
11. T	11. C
12. T	12. N
13. T	13. K
14. F	14. A
15. T	15. J

Fill-Ins

1. 60 mph
2. Ha ha ha
3. Yuk yuk; oye oye; har har; he he, jaa jaa; eeeya eeyaa; aah aah
4. Enthusiasm
5. Ease stress; lessen anger; kick-start joy; enhance creativity; lift your spirits; cause others to laff, gain attention
6. Stickers; collages; posters; happy paper plates; bookmarks

7. Halls and walls
8. You too
9. Hairstyle
10. Moss-Cess Process
11. Stickers
12. Dr. Norman Cousins
13. Label
14. Alaska
15. World

List of Relevant Resources

The following items are grouped by topic and serve as references related to information discussed in *The Enthusiasm–Laffter Connection.*

Enthusiasm:

Kimbro, Dennis. *Think and Grow Rich: A Black Choice.* New York: Fawcett, 1992.

Meadows, Mike. "Enthusiasm in the Workplace." *IBM Newsletter*, Tucson edition, September 1992.

Carlock, LaNetta. "How to Motivate Todays' Students." *Journal of American Association of Medical Assistants.*

Hughes, Langston, *Selected Poems of Langston Hughes, "Mother to Son."* New York, Vintage Books, 1974.

Laffter and Gelotology:

Cousins, Norman. *Anatomy of an Illness.* New York: Bantam Doubleday Dell, 1981.

Brody, Robert. "Anatomy of a Laff." *American Health.* November/ December, 1983.

Olona, Mary. "Going From Serious To Fun, and Still Remaining Professional." *Journal of Counseling and Development* (October 1988).

Finley, Leigh. "Laughter." *San Diego Union.* March 11, 1984.

Hicks, John, and Dan Jordan. *First Responders Handbook of Humor.* Santa Clarita, CA: Quiet Man Publishing, 2006.

Quinion, Michael. "Gelotologist." *World Wide Words.* June 2006.

von Rooyen, Smuts. "Gelotology 101 for Christmas." *Grace Unconditional.* Summer 2002.

Traywick, LaVona. "Health Notes: Humor, Laughter and Aging." *Rural Arkansas*. January 2009.

Nabbefield, Joe. "Guru of Laughter Pays Therapeutic Visit." *La Jolla Light*. July 19, 1984.

Southwestern College Health Services Newsletter. "Healthy Heart Beat." 2001.

AARP Health Care Options Newsletter. "F.Y.I., Laugh Your Way to Better Health." July 2001.

Visualization:

Waas, Lane Longino. *Imagine That!* Fawnskin, CA: Jalmar Press, 1991.

Maltz, Maxwell. *Psychocybernetics*. New York: Simon & Schuster, 1960.

Kryder, Ralph. "Shoptalk." *Sports Illustrated*, June 6, 1983.

Frederick, Bruce. "The That's It Response." *Journal of Health, Physical Education, & Recreation* (April 1972).

Just, Sheri, and Carolyn Flynn. *The Complete Idiot's Guide to Creative Visualization*. New York: Alpha Books, 2005.

Further Acknowledgements

Bob "Hubba Jubba" Moss was absolutely the best of my hires while establishing the physical education department at UCSD. I have never seen anybody more full of the "did its" than Bob Moss. **Dr. Ted Forbes,** retired physical education department chair at UCSD. Bob Moss is the most creative person I have ever met. **Dr. Jack Douglass,** retired UC San Diego administrator/faculty member. I know no other educator who possesses a greater passion for sharing enthusiasm than Bob Moss! **Dr. Alfred Arrington,** retired UA Pine Bluff administrator. Bob was ahead of the rest of the country in his teaching. His passion for being an innovative methodologist overcame ridicule and disbelief by many, and we know the things he forwarded have significant merit and content. **Dr. Bert Kobayashi,** retired physical education department at UCSD. Through the years, Bob has not wavered from his dynamic style of laughter as a means for gaining and maintaining positive attitudes. I am struck by his unique style of sharing his world of laughter with others. **Dr. Stan Butler,** kinesiology faculty member, San Jose State University.

In my many years working with Bob, he is one of the most inspirational persons in my life. He makes moments special and leaves a legacy of laughter and enthusiasm to everyone he touches. **Gary Zerecky,** retired basketball coach and current faculty member at De Anza Community College. Bob's optimistic and contagious outlook was a positive source of inspiration for our multicultural group and entire membership. **Belinda Rector,** physical education teacher and past president of California's professional physical education teacher's organization. Bob Moss and I thrived on efforts to successfully increase the numbers of awards and leadership roles achieved by our multicultural colleagues at all levels of our professional physical educator's organization. **John Payne,** physical education faculty member, Evergreen College and past president of California's professional physical education teacher's organization. Moss's belief in laughter, positive thinking and enthusiasm is contagious and I caught it hook line and sinker. He has set out to change the world one laugh at a time. **Carmi Strom,** school principal, San Diego, California.

Bob Moss's gift of laughter transcends generations. He is one of the most genuine persons on our planet. **Tim White,** teacher and coach, Julian High School. Hubba Jubba's teaching enthusiasm and expertise has had a very positive influence on me. I have become more creative while emulating Bob's unique style. His dedication to students and the teaching profession is second to none. **Jeff Woodland,** physical education teacher, San Diego. I had the pleasure to watch Bob Moss fill an auditorium of hesitant, unsure students with love, enth-u-u-siasm and laffter. He showed the students how to tap into their natural abilities. **Mike Love,** math teacher and his school District's 2010 teacher of the year. Bob Moss's unique brand of enthusiasm and laughter has had a profound effect on my teaching career, since attending his in-service presentation back in 1980. Many of the things I learned that day I still apply in my classrooms today. **Stan Murphy,** teacher, San Diego HS and national teacher of the year finalist in 2005. As a student athlete at UC San Diego, I was introduced to Bob Moss's motivation concepts. Now, 27 years later, his work has been validated by research in neuroscience and psychology affirming what he knew then. I continue to be inspired by him and teach my athletes the values he taught me. **Carin Crawford,** San Diego State University water polo coach. Bob Moss focuses on enthusiasm as a key to how we see and enjoy life. Bob's book is an easy read for those desiring to possess a more positive outlook on life. **Leonard Burnett,** Orlando, Florida radio personality and business owner.

I have used Bob's motivational techniques to have fun and maintain a positive attitude throughout my career. He has been and continues to be a mentor of greatness to so many people, and his unique legacy shines in all folks he influences. **John "J.C." Crouch,** former baseball executive and now business person in Kauai, Hawaii. Bob Moss has been my friend and mentor since I was in junior high school. During that time he taught me imagery techniques to improve my athletic and umpiring skills. I cherish the fact I was able to instill his concepts in the lives of my now adult children. **David Shively,** soft-wear products administrator, Freemont, California. I was the NCAA basketball scoring leader in my freshman year, and then transferred to UC San Diego where I met Bob Moss. He has made me a better father, husband and teacher to those I supervise. **John Saintignon,** professional basketball coach/consultant, Orange County, California.

"Hubba Jubba" Moss can get a deep belly laugh out of the grumpiest subject. While a student at UC San Diego, he instilled in me the confidence, humility and enthusiasm to become successful at everything I do! **Ian Altman,** protégé of the Moss-Cess Process, bestselling author, international speaker and sales advisor, Washington, D.C.. Bob Moss's unique approach to teaching the use of laughter, visualization and positive mind sets assisted my son to be selected in the 2011 Major League Baseball draft. I have watched him encourage many student athletes to successfully compete in sports, graduate and then assume quality leadership endeavors in their representative fields. **James Matz,** award winning mega realtor, Chicago, Illinois. Some 30 years ago, my softball team took our games very-very seriously. We enjoyed watching Moss's enthusiastic and entertaining umpire skills. We thank him for always reminding us softball was just a game and to have fun while playing it. **Mike "Motor City" Allen,** former ASA softball player. Coach Moss, my high school football coach some 45 years ago, inspired me and my teammates to achieve successful leadership roles in our later career endeavors. I can never thank him enough for the valuable attitudes he instilled in me. **James Tucker,** Mission Bay HS class of 1967.

A person who definitely had a major impact on me during my college career was Bob Moss. His dynamic and friendly mentoring not only benefited my physical (baseball) skills, but helped mold me into a better man outside of the game too. **Lloyd Burchett,** UA Pine Bluff 2011 graduate. "Hubba Jubba" Moss and I were umpiring partners working at least 100 games a season for some 20 years. We were legendary figures in an activity where game officials are rarely praised for the work they do. What a joy it was to work with Hubba Jubba; I never worked with a better umpire or had finer friend. **Pat McDonald,** retired umpire and newspaper associate, San Diego, California. Thank you Bob Moss for your assistance and support at our Youth Education through Sports (YES Program), during the 1999 NCAA water polo clinic at UC San Diego. Your ability to relate to over 300 participants was not only effective, but enjoyable to watch, and your enthusiastic approach was wonderful. **Tony Mason** and **Rochelle Collins,** NCAA Y.E.S. program coordinators.

Printed in the United States
By Bookmasters

THE MELTING OF THE
GOLDEN SPOON

THE MELTING OF THE
GOLDEN SPOON

GETTING BACK THE MIDDLE CLASS

Michael E. Mitzelfelt

authorHOUSE®

AuthorHouse™
1663 Liberty Drive
Bloomington, IN 47403
www.authorhouse.com
Phone: 1-800-839-8640

Published by AuthorHouse   04/12/2012

ISBN:978-1-4678-0300-7 (sc)
ISBN: 978-1-4678-0301-4 (e)

Library of Congress Control Number: 2011919466

Any people depicted in stock imagery provided by Thinkstock are models, and such images are being used for illustrative purposes only.
Certain stock imagery © Thinkstock.

This book is printed on acid-free paper.

Because of the dynamic nature of the Internet, any web addresses or links contained in this book may have changed since publication and may no longer be valid. The views expressed in this work are solely those of the author and do not necessarily reflect the views of the publisher, and the publisher hereby disclaims any responsibility for them.

Dedication

This book is dedicated to my friends and family and the co-workers
that HAVE stuck by me. I have a special place in my heart for the
chosen people who put my feelings first above their own. This is
what life is about and they will be rewarded someday. They are
the type of people that will lead to make a difference. The rest will
learn that their own greed is no better than the people stealing
from their pocket. This is something you can't teach you either
think of others or you don't. It is also dedicated to the elderly,
veterans, and the people who try to make a living and struggle to
pay the bills. We are all in the same boat and I hope you know now
you are not alone. I will continue to work to get the word out that
we have had enough. I will watch attentively to see
who is listening.

CHAPTER 1

Well there is so much to say and so little time to say it so let us start from the beginning. I come from a small town in Central Illinois called Manito. I know it is a funny name but it actually derives from an Indian name I am told, as the town began in the Sand Ridge state forest near the famous Goofy Ridge, Illinois. Yes I said Goofy Ridge, a very small community that was rumored to be a hide out for Al Capone in the early days. The crime rate in this little town is outrageous for the number of people that live there. Basically there is no law to keep things in order so sometimes things get a little out of hand, a murder here, a beating there, typical hick town. Manito was moved from the state forest to a location closer to the thriving railroad during that period. This is the place I went to school growing up and my stomping grounds so to speak.

I started out life living in between Goofy Ridge and Manito actually living in the state forest. We were pretty poor as I remember in a little house of which I shared a bedroom with my two brothers and sister. I remember pictures of me taking baths in the kitchen sink if you can believe that or not. We never had much, junky cars that barely ran and a billy goat in the front yard that I hated. That goat got his kicks by bucking me around like a ping pong ball whenever I went outside. MAN I DESPISED THAT FREAKING GOAT! Our car never had a muffler because the roads were so bad it would just rip em off as fast as my dad could wire it up. The biggest thrill in those parts was watching the local museum dig for Indian artifacts in front of the house. I was a happy kid though even though we were dirt poor. Our meals always included bisquick and that powdered milk that made you puke. On occasion we would have some spam and if we were lucky somebody we knew butchered so we got some real meat now and then.

The reason we were so poor wasn't that my parents were lazy which is what you might be thinking. My dad fell at work at a power plant and pretty much broke every bone in his body. He was never supposed to be able to function after that but he was a tough man. I remember my brothers telling me when they brought him home if you entered the bed room he would yelp from the vibration of the floor boards flexing and the bed moving. It was a bad scene but slowly he got better. Of course where he worked would not pay for anything so he hired a lawyer so we wouldn't starve. Back then just like today, it was common place for a lawyer to be paid off. This turned out to be the case and my dad received NOTHING. Still we managed to scrape by and later he found another job with, I will call it Big Yellow, one of the biggest and best employers in the area. Things started to look up and begin to change.

At the age of 5 my dad decided to build a house closer to Manito on five acres of land. It was built on sand and I remember you couldn't walk without a sock and shoelaces full of sandburs. But it was a way bigger house and with six people we sure needed the space. Our first day there I was playing in the sandburs with the only toy I had, an old Tonka dump truck. I tootled along making truck noises and pushed right into a big ol' hog nose snake. Talk about scaring the life out of a five year old kid! I didn't go outside for a while after that. But it was still nice having some room to move. And we were a lot happier as a family getting a few things here and there. Dad was in a union and had a little stability, it was like a whole new world for us.

My dad was a very hard working, stern man who came from a large family. His dad died from leukemia before I was born, and I never had the pleasure of meeting my grandpa. My grandpa worked in a foundry and was a strong dude. I saw pictures of him he looked kind of mean and had arms like cannons. They weren't the kind of arms you see today, steroid injected freaks. They were hard work arms and were very impressive. He became very sick though and withered down to nothing and my dad had to work through high school to help support the family. My mom, bless her heart, did his homework and helped him graduate. I am assuming my dad got his hard ass traits through my grandpa and it was in the genes. His whole family was basically a band of brothers with a couple girls, they stuck together and didn't back down from anyone. They were ruthless from what I saw and the stories I have been told.

I remember him coming home on many an occasion a bloody freakin mess from getting into with somebody. He and his brother got the bright idea to get into it with a bunch of bikers who flipped them off, they showed up with gravel in their faces covered in blood. BUT THEY WERE GIGGLING ABOUT IT! This was their idea of a good time as odd as that sounds. He and his brothers of course loved to drink and that probably escalated a few of these situations. But the bottom line is he came from a line of some tough hombres. He tried to instill being tough to us kids as a passed down to generation kind of thing.

A day at the house never went by without some type of work to be done. I was young and stupid and the baby of the family so he left me alone for the most part. I was smart enough to claim ignorance and stay away from him as much as possible. My brothers though were not so fortunate. They had to plant fence post around five acres of pasture one by one with a shovel, not a post hole digger. It took them about 6 months and they complained about it every day. He would check their progress daily and if enough didn't get done there was hell to pay. He would let them have it and have it good. If there was an easier way to do it, so what, they weren't going to do it that way. Man I felt sorry for them but as I said I stayed out of it. It was my only defense.

As I got older he kind of started to crack the whip on me a little bit, not near like my brothers, but he started to instill these values into my bloodstream. I was a pretty good kid for the most part and I never got the beatings my brothers did but I remember a few. Two in particular ring a bell. I was sick and in bed and I THOUGHT my dad had left for work. My brothers being in high school and rock and roll gurus, had the stereo cranked up. They too had thought dad went to work. We were all wrong as my mom was not home to run interference as she often did to save our lives. I wasn't feeling good and the music blaring was starting to get on my nerves. I screamed at the top of my lungs "TURN OFF THE RADIO"!!! This did not work as my brothers rarely listened to what I said. I began to get ill-tempered just like my dad and yelled again only this time "TURN OFF THE DAMN RADIO"!! And just like the first time I got no response. Finally I began screaming "TURN OFF THAT F n RADIO" as loud as I could yell it. I yelled it over and over to no avail. Then I decided to look in the doorway as I decided to turn my head instead of yelling at the ceiling. There he was, the glare cut me in half. I don't remember much after that as he yanked me out of that bed and literally destroyed me. I tried the I'M SICK line of defense it was all I had since mom was not there to defend me. You know I found out that this had no bearing on the current situation. I learned very quickly that nine year olds should not engage in this type of language. It took years to recover from that beating.

The other time was when I came from school and noticed dad laying in the bed as he did not go to work that day. My dad rarely missed work so I knew something was up. I asked my mom why dad was home and she kind of grinned. She said don't worry about it and go do something just stay away from him. She was locked up like she was being interrogated about the Kennedy assassination. I was stupid and just had to know why she grinned and would tell me nothing about what was going on. She started dinner so I crept ever so slowly into dad's room. He was rolled over on his side away from me so I couldn't see his face. He heard me and told me to get out without looking at me. By this time I was overrun with ignorance, I WAS NOT GOING TO LEAVE THAT ROOM WITHOUT ANSWERS! This was a huge mistake I would later discover. I asked him if he was sick and why he wasn't at work. Like a hissing rattlesnake he gave warning a second time. I didn't listen as he told me to get out again as a courtesy to save me. I was persistent like a car salesman and invited death like a moron. I walked around to the other side of the bed slowly and finally found my answer. His mouth was swelled up like a gorilla! He looked like Fred Flintstone only worse! I started laughing my ass off as any witty human would. HOLY ****! That ol' boy shot up out of that bed like Jessie Owens and proceeded to . . . try to console me, yeah that's it. (That is what I am supposed to say) This was a very embarrassed and angry individual. Two things you didn't do are tell my dad to shut up or laugh at him I learned through experience. After my intense beating and hysterical sobbing I learned that he ate garlic and had an allergic reaction to it. That was all mom had to say. Sometimes I think she wanted me to find out for myself. From now on I heeded her advice on such matters.

Now if I were reading this I would assume my father was an abusive, evil, individual. The fact is he was a great man. He was mean and gruff on the outside but very giving. I remember us delivering a milk cow to my uncle for his birthday because he was poor for the most part. Countless people borrowed money off of him and I never knew if he got paid back. I would venture to say probably not. Things were different when I was a kid, a beating was not translated into abuse. If we kids had it coming we got it as per offense. Something minor would include an increase in work load or your typical grounding, more severe offenses including a lashing of some sort. But let's face it as a kid you are aware of what you are doing and there are consequences if you do it. Nowadays there are no consequences for actions, Kids will blame it on their uncle who gave them black licorice instead of the red they wanted. Society changed when parents were no longer able to punish kids the way they were taught.

Finally they gave up punishing them at all. Punishment leads to bad behavior now, and bad behavior has no responsibility in the equation. This has seemed to be the biggest lesson I learned in life from my parents. You do something to hurt someone or something you get it back, sometimes twice as bad as you give it. Things sure have changed.

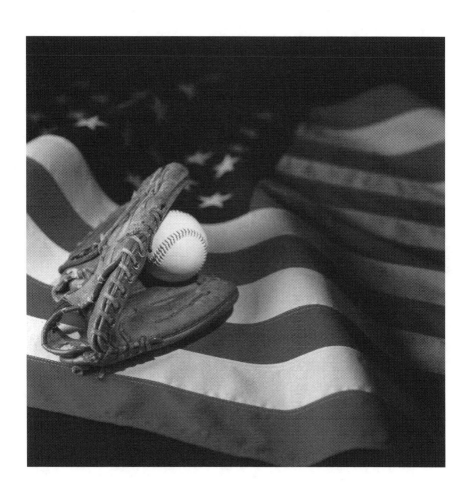

CHAPTER 2

As a kid growing up we had three basic channels on the TV. Wasn't a whole lot to do unless you enjoyed being outside. And with limited funds as a kid you had to be creative to find something to pass the time. We would grab those round sleds and use them as shields to fight with walnuts. Being young and mentally challenged we failed to see the danger in this activity. Now if you have ever lived in the woods you know how hard these walnuts are. Even with that stinky, green, cushion on the outside one could indeed kill you if it hit you in the right spot. Nevertheless it was one of our favorite pastimes with me and the neighbors. We would pick teams build dirt mounds for bunkers and begin fighting as soon as someone screamed an obscenity. It was fun being in battle with teammates even if you couldn't stand the kids on your side. Things would start off innocently enough with a few plinks here and there. But eventually someone is gonna get hit and the real fight is on from this point. There was always supposed to be a boundary line we were all supposed to adhere to but as soon as a wound was opened all bets were off. Once the anger of being struck kicked in the cheating also began. Someone would cross the line and fire one of these rock hard grenades from ten feet or less. As you can probably guess this is when someone was seriously split open or knocked on their butt. The manliness was now a thing of the past and the wussiness kicked in. There was usually screaming, name calling, and of course sobbing. No one could blame the poor sap though we were smart enough to know it hurt and glad it wasn't us. But the bad part was we couldn't let the injury leak out to our parents. After a period of time, when cooler heads prevailed we would band together. If we told the truth the true enjoyment of this event would be no longer so we had to do what kids do . . . LIE! We would always come up with something and oddly enough the parent would believe it. Later on in life I wondered if they really bought it or just didn't have enough evidence to prosecute.

Unfortunately one of the kids in that story had a tragic death. It was always his house that we had these fun times at. We remained friends over the years as he moved away and chatted from time to time. He turned out to be kind of a wild sort, but he kind of was wild as a kid too. He from what I hear had a little too much to drink after a night at the bar. He put something on the stove and proceeded to pass out on the couch. Of course one thing led to another and the upstairs apartment he lived in caught fire. He wasn't coherent enough to wake up and ended up being badly burned and passing away in the blaze. His dad came to the scene of the fire and had a heart attack. He also died instantly that night, what a sad ending to a lot of good times. Things like that make you think of how quick it can happen.

The other things we engaged in at that age were sports. Mainly baseball was the sport of choice. I absolutely loved the game of baseball, I CRAVED IT. I would be outside until dark with a tennis ball throwing it off the side of the house. Dad would get mad because I would rub a big bare spot in the yard where I pitched from. He knew how much I loved it though and didn't pursue it, just bitched about it occasionally. At least this activity kept me out of trouble for the most part. I was a huge St. Louis Cardinals fan at that age. My brother was and he threatened me if I wasn't as well. I was a big fan of Lou Brock in particular. Things weren't like they are today with cable television. Now every game is televised with a lot of hype in between. We had three opportunities to watch a ball game if we were lucky. Who could forget Monday night baseball on ABC with Earl Weaver, Don Drysdale, and Jim Palmer? Oh how I loved Monday night baseball. You also had the game of the week on NBC with Joe Garagiola and Tony Kubek. And if it were a clear day you could pick up a Cardinal game on Sunday on a channel from Springfield. This was on a crappy television with snow all over it, tin foil caked on the antenna for better reception. Did this ever really work? Other than that I would be camped out in front of the radio every night listening to Jack Buck and playing the game in my mind. You know looking back I think that is why I loved the game so much, you had to use your imagination with it. As a kid your imagination is a key part of everything. There was no instant replay, no pitch tracker, none of that crap. Just my radio and my mind is all I needed.

You don't know how many world series were won in my back yard, damn near one every day. In my mind I was on the mound for that pivotal game. No one gave me a chance but they didn't know the stuff I had. The crowd was in my head, I could hear them but no one else could. I would take a gander around once in a while to make sure no one was watching me from across the road or through a window. They would think I was crazy or abused these days. There's that abuse thing again! If no one was watching I would even mumble a little play by play just loud enough for only me to hear it. I would have a spot on the wall I had to hit for a strike anywhere else was a ball. I would usually play the Cubs because I hated them. Even though in real life there was no way they could play in a world series because they were in the same league I loved knocking the Cubs off. On occasion I would play the Yankees because everyone hated the Yankees back then too. I would usually come in to close the deal in the ninth inning, I could hear the fans cheering me when I walked to the mound. I always pretended I had never pitched in a major league game and the manager took a chance on me. (yeah, like that would happen) I would promptly hit the first batter because I enjoyed that, probably because I was beaten as a child. Then I would walk the next two to make it interesting. I could hear the fans getting torqued off in my mind and chants of "GET HIM OUT OF THERE"!! This only made me more focused and intense. I would strike out the next two batters on six pitches with the hard stuff. The fans attitude now started to change a little once they saw the gas I could bring. It was all up to this, bases loaded, two outs, up by one run. I could hear Mike Shannon saying it in my head, "OL ABNER HAS DONE IT AGAIN FOLKS"!! I would throw three consecutive balls and the fans would get restless and a few boos would arise. I took some time and wipe my brow, positioned my hat, and took a deep breath before returning to the bald spot in the grass. I would fire two consecutive blazing fastballs for strikes as the hitter looked up in the air in frustration. If the pitch was really a ball I would claim it was a foul ball and continue. Then I would rise up and blow a heater right past him for the third strike. The fans would go crazy as I ran in to meet the catcher, but I had to keep cool in case people were looking, maybe go behind a tree to celebrate. I remember almost coming to tears at times. And that's how I won a world series in my back yard.

I played baseball every single day in some way. I played little league, Jr. High, and High School baseball. Later on I coached an adult league, Pony league, and even High School ball. I just could not believe how the mentality of this game has changed. Maybe it was the inner toughness my dad had instilled in me, who knows. Kids nowadays are the biggest candy asses for the most part I have ever seen. When I lost a game I took it personally and didn't like it at all. Nowadays parents want you to reward for failure and accept it as a regular part of life. When I coach I like to teach a few of life's lessons in between to try to make the kids successful in things they choose to do later on. I have learned this is forbidden in today's society. Once again it is considered abusive to get on a kid for not trying or sit him on the bench. Even if a kid throws a bat or curses it is not his fault. You are supposed to give them a shoulder to cry on and tell them it's ok. I have two words for that BULL *   *   *! I'm not talking about that kid who has no talent and gives it everything, I love those kids. I am speaking of those spoiled kids who have the most expensive of everything, are fed from the golden spoon, and don't have to work cause they are already good enough. I just can't handle that, it drives me crazy. I wasn't like this I just tried and tried hard. I expect that from my players and when I don't get it? That word, consequence. Everybody loses, it is a fact of life, but you don't have to accept it for everything you do. That message has gone down the toilet I am afraid. Encouragement is a great tool for coaching but when you expect it at all times it is no longer valid. Eventually every kid has to stand on his own two feet and accept accountability for how he or she performs. It makes them a better person in the long run.

I agreed to coach the High School freshman/sophomore team and this is a perfect example of what I am referring to. These kids were not very good and not expected to win. Being from a small town, I only had enough to field a team. I had my work cut out for me but I thought maybe the way I did things would turn things around. I had some really good kids on that team and I had some that could care less. Of course I took a lot of time with the kids that wanted to get better, I could see a little of me in them I guess. We started winning some games. We beat a team by the ten run rule on a Thursday and played extremely well. I was so proud of those kids at the time. We played the same team four days later and got beat 16 to 2. I was absolutely livid because these kids showed from the start they flat out didn't care and gave up. I chewed them good and told them they should be ashamed of the effort they gave and that their parents drove an hour to watch it. They should apologize to their parents for not trying and wasting their time. In the middle of my conversation a parent interrupts me and tells me I have to cut my talk short. They have cookies and drinks ready for the kids. Need I say more? That is what is wrong with society today in a nutshell. You can agree to disagree but prove me wrong. How can anyone achieve when rewarded for effortless failure? It cannot work that way and we have to change it.

It is even worse at the lower levels. The kids do not show up for practice and expect to play over a kid that has been sweating, learning, and paying his debt to be better. The parents give me nasty little talks of how little Jimmy isn't playing and he isn't happy. When little Jimmy isn't happy the parents aren't happy. The reason little Jimmy sat on the bench is because little Jimmy decided swimming was more important than the commitment to his team. Tyler on the other hand showed up for practice, stayed after practice, and is playing instead of Jimmy. Who is wrong here? And the parents who don't want to coach because they don't want the responsibility have the nerve to question how you do it. When you are VOLUNTEERING because no one else will do it! My dad who worked second shift didn't make it to many of my games as a kid but he made a few. He did not interfere other than kicking me in the butt to try harder. I remember one game I struck out on a called third strike and I said something smart to the umpire. He was waiting for me in the dugout with that LOOK. He asked me if I wanted to keep playing and I said yes. He proceeded to order me to apologize to the umpire or he was yanking my ass to the car. I walked up apologized and shook the umpires hand and said I just got frustrated. He laughed and said that was ok buddy. My dad walked back and sat down, that was the end of it. I learned a valuable lesson that day of how the game should be played, and how it should be coached. Respect the game because you won't be able to play it forever.

I finally retired from playing baseball at the age of 41, and retired from coaching as well. The way things are today I just can't adapt to the new style of play. I like to call this, pardon my French, the candy ass way. I see it in the major leagues worse than ever. What ever happened to playing for the love of the game? I realize you have to love it in some way to play 162 games or more a year but only if you get paid to love it. I see players not running out ground balls, not hustling, and not appreciating the fans who pay big money to see them not care. It never used to be that way, what happened? It is what happens when you eat out of that golden spoon I referred to earlier. The little things don't matter anymore, only the money. Who cares that a guy putting in 60 hours a week spends half his paycheck to take his kids to a ballgame. These kids look up to a player as a hero. How does a hero thank a kid who worships him? Make his dad pay nine dollars for a beer, six dollars for a hot dog, and six dollars for a coke. That is gratitude isn't it. Listen up owners I'm talking about you too. You are just as disgusting because as a part of corporate America you would still charge it even if you didn't pay these ridiculous salaries. Quit hiding behind it as you do during every labor dispute. I know players, and not just baseball, are part of labor unions of which I am fully in favor of. But labor unions were not organized to promote this type of fleecing of the general public. They were designed to produce FAIR wages, health benefits, and safe working conditions for workers. Why do I never hear this brought up? Where are these million dollar players to lend a helping hand to their fellow union brothers and sisters. Instead of walking side by side with the people who created their opportunities many years ago they turn their back. They hold out for more money because 200 million just isn't enough. They have to provide for their families you know. How soon the little guys are forgotten, the one's fighting to keep their family under a roof. I just don't see the big picture from a millionaires eyes.

CHAPTER 3

My father was a very big union advocate as he worked in a Foundry stated earlier. The guy came home with burns on him as he was a maintenance welder and worked hard for 30 years. He became ill from an occupational disease which cut his working career short. Basically I watched him wither away and die just like his father. As a union worker my dad didn't expect to get rich but he did expect to be able to provide for his family for his efforts. This is something every worker in my mind has a right to as long as he is providing a service. I understand there are small businesses that can't afford to pay people but would if they could. It is the major corporations that feed the top WITH THE GOLDEN SPOON, make millions, and even billions, that make me sick. They do not care whether a guy can't pay for his kid's surgery, put food on the table, or pay the light bill. What is wrong with this country? I don't have to go into detail about the "recession for us, but not for them" we just went through. We saw a lot of billionaires made then didn't we? And millions of people out of work with nowhere to turn. This was just another ploy to eliminate the middle class who is now lower class.

My dad went on strike a few times during my childhood and those were extremely tough times. I was too young to know what was really going on for the most part but I sure do now. They went on strike because they did not want a two tier wage system. Which means a young kid would come in and make about half the wage of the guy he is working side by side with. This is a common ploy by corporate America to create two classes, very rich, and very poor. This was a way to get the ball rolling to take away other benefits later on down the road. And more importantly it was an attempt to bust the union or at least get a good start on it. I remember everyone calling my dad and the strikers greedy without really taking a look at what was going on. The media of course portrays the union workforce as being greedy without putting all the facts out there. And they always hand pick the most unintellectual and unintelligent person they can find to interview. And I am sure that is purely accident.

I am sure there are greedy guys out there only trying to get more money but I have to say from my own experience that an overwhelming majority is out there trying to keep a future for the next generation. Trying to make sure they can keep food on the table for people, reasonable health benefits, and pensions for people so they can retire before they die. What in the world is wrong with that? And who buys the cars? Who supports local business? And who pays the taxes? The people who are losing everything are the ones that pay for everything. These are all questions that aren't asked when evaluating labor disputes. It is a one sided portrayal in my opinion. We have to keep these things for our children and grandchildren. People now are starting to understand it wasn't all about greed. Look what happened in Wisconsin with the state workers. It is now so widespread it affects everyone, every state, every business. The top gets richer and richer, there is no middle, and the lower gets poorer and poorer. Back when I was a kid people flew that American flag with pride. We were the greatest country on earth! Now we are the most crooked country on earth, and the greediest thanks to corporate America. I am sure there is someone out there calling me a communist, a rich person no doubt. I am proud of where I came from but not so proud of what my country represents now. I am proud of the men and women who defend this country for our freedom. I am not proud of the country that puts them in that position for foreign oil and treats them like dirt when they get home. I am sure this makes sense if you really think about it. I am proud of the people who work every day to a dismal future. I am not proud of the people who created the dismal future and continue to profit from it. How could anyone be proud of what this country has turned into? I keep hearing it's just the way things are. I don't accept that.

CHAPTER 4

As a kid you always hear your parents and grandparents talk about the "good ol' days." Now I am talking about them. This means two things, I am getting old, and every generation is getting worse as it goes. My translation of good ol' days means that everything you did back then wasn't a pain in the ass like it is today. Every year that goes by the world becomes more technical, more automated, and more time consuming. Automation is supposed to make things easier we are told, but we all know it is just another way the golden spoon feeds itself. I know there are a lot of people if not everyone feeling my pain. This is just another way to pad some pockets and keep from paying a real live human to help us with our issues and make our lives easier. Somebody is always out to screw you and automation makes it so much easier to accomplish this.

Whatever happened to talking to people, a personality on the other end of the line. An automated voice has no compassion, no reasoning, no anything. And if you are lucky enough to speak to a live person you are most likely going to get someone from India that you cannot understand. This is just another fine example of corporate greed at work. Why give you service you can understand when you can pay someone a quarter of the wage and hopefully you will get mad and hang up. Problem solved! I had an issue with a credit card about a month ago when I received my bill. It appeared that someone had gotten ahold of my credit card number and charged over a thousand dollars on it. After being enraged I called the card company. Already steaming I receive the automation we all love so much. It was so cool having all these options, about 15 minutes worth, of course none that I actually needed. Finally I find the option and get ahold of a person. The line was static I could hardly hear anything and I get a foreigner to boot. I could not understand a word this person said and became increasingly angry as time went on. I finally asked for a supervisor and low and behold another person from India! I could pick up every other word this time so this was a keeper! After a half an hour of translation I learned someone used my credit card number to purchase online classes learning of all things the English language. I explained I obviously already knew the English language so therefore why would I spend a thousand dollars to learn it? They made me contact the company that the classes were purchased through. Great service huh. So I now go through the same routine and finally get through to someone. You guessed it, another person from India, and the accent and connection are even worse than the first person I talked to at the credit card company. After an hour or so I have both parties on speaker phone at the same time. And to make things easier on me they both start speaking the language of their preference so I have no chance of eavesdropping. I have no idea what is being said and after stewing for about 15 minutes I butt in and say are we about finished here? They pretty much forgot I was even there. This ordeal took about 2 hours and I got nothing accomplished. All I wanted was someone I could understand! I am not blaming the worker they were just doing their job to the best of their ability. They would have every right to be angry if the shoe was on the other foot and I was getting calls from India and answering their questions in English. Needless to say it took a month or better and me threatening cancellation of all services to get something done. Do you think they went through this type of thing in the good ol' days?

The bad part is they will screw you locally too not just globally. I had a hospital visit that cost a significant amount of money. I received the bill and wanted to make payments because I didn't have the money to pay it all at once. No dice they sent it to collections immediately. I couldn't understand why the hospital billing would ruin my credit because I couldn't pay thousands of dollars up front. I was willing to pay for everything just needed to do it monthly. It didn't matter, the new American way. So the collection agency gets it and I start making payments. I worked a bunch of overtime, saved every penny I could and paid off the last 1600 dollars. I get a phone call a month later and ask why I haven't been making payments and I explained that I paid it off a month ago. They say we have no record of that sir you still owe 1600 dollars. I became absolutely enraged I said I would get a cancelled check and show that I paid it. They couldn't accept that, I was either to pay it or they would take me to court. I said fine take me to court I had the proof I paid it. No way that they were going to get another 1600 dollars out of me, no way. So I am all ready to go to court and don't hear anything for another month. Then I get a letter saying I didn't show up for court so the plaintiff won the case. I was court ordered to pay them the money. I called the courthouse and asked what had happened and they explained I had been given a summons on a Sunday to appear. I explained I had not been presented a summons at any time. They had a date and the guy that supposedly gave it to me. I lived alone so no chance anyone else could have received it either. I asked if they had my signature that I received it. They explained they didn't need a signature. THEN HOW DO YOU KNOW I RECEIVED IT?? Tough, guess who had to pay another 1600 dollars even though he had proof he paid it? That's right good ol' me. Working people don't have a fighting chance in this country anymore. And it is only getting worse my friends.

Back when I was a kid in the good or days people that I knew only used credit cards if they absolutely had to. Now it is just another example of corporate America taking advantage of a desperate society. I know some people live beyond their means and abuse them but I don't think that is where the problem lies. People aren't using them for vacations anymore they are using them to pay the light bill and basic life necessities. That is why it is sickening when I see people knee deep in credit card debt when they were only trying to take care of their family. What else are they supposed to do? They can't pay their bills so they have to use them. Survival is a terrible situation to be in but millions of people in the greatest country on earth are in that predicament. Why? They don't make enough money to survive. I have heard well to do people say people in that situation have to learn to do without things. They can do without internet and cell phones. How is someone supposed to stay current in today's society without internet? How can they find a better paying job if they aren't current? How many jobs require cell phones that are willing to pay anything? And how are kids supposed to keep up with the others in school without internet? This is easier said than done golden spooners. The only way people can keep up with technology is if they have it. You have to have money to have it. Less and less people have the money to pay for it. They are in a no win situation and it is going to continue to divide the class of people. More and more will drop out as they will not be able to continue financially to keep up. Who benefits from this? Think about it.

Things were so much easier when people made money, enjoyed their jobs, had a mom at home to take care of the kids like I did. Where did all of that go? Well it doesn't take a genius to figure out the money is still out there it's just going into a few pockets instead of a bunch. Mom can't stay at home unless she is on state aid which means other people are watching their kids. What kind of values can a parent teach in a couple of hours a day. The weekends used to be for fun, not anymore. The parents are either working to put a little extra food on the table, or they are knee deep trying to keep up with what they didn't get done during the week. Who suffers from all this? The American family is splitting up right before our very eyes and no one cares. Kids are more distant from their parents and running amuck. They don't have the guidance they used to, the parents have little or no time to deal with them and they take advantage of it. Any kid would if given the opportunity. I have seen the change just by coaching these kids, who knows what happens outside the ball field. I think we see it every day in the papers to answer that question.

When I was a kid my cousins would come over and we would play baseball or board games. The parents would just sit and visit for hours until we tuckered out. On the weekends we would all pile in the car and head down to the lake and go fishing. There was always some sort of family thing going on, whether it was a fish fry or just hanging out we always spent time with families. We didn't need lavish trips to have a good time, just good ol' family fun in the good ol' days. Now that most of my family has passed on I never see anyone. Everyone is too busy including me. The only time I see anyone is if someone dies and that is sad. People don't have time to value the family anymore. Today everyone works longer hours for half the pay. They don't have enough hours in the day to influence the lives of their children. I really would love to see the greatest country in the world rise up and give us these things back. But you know who is going to fight it every step of the way. And then question why society is the way it is. Why is the crime rate so high? Why do people snap and go into offices firing? Why don't parents keep an eye on their kids to prevent another columbine? Man what horrible parents, they must have been. Amazing isn't it? Like I said it doesn't take a genius to figure it out. More pressure, less time, less money, equals instability somewhere down the line.

I remember a time when people were proud of where they worked. They would brag about it and talk about it for hours. I can't remember the last time I heard someone say they loved their job without giggling with sarcasm after they said it. What the hell happened in between those years? I know it is those greedy workers, well I think we know now that is not the case. It starts at the top, not the bottom, and as soon as everyone is on the same page we have a shred of hope of getting our lives back. Until then, only God can help us.

CHAPTER 5

I have shared my views with you in the prior chapters of what is wrong with this country and I am not done yet, not even close. I know many people have experienced the same frustrations and same thoughts but are never articulated. I have spoken ill of this country but there are so many good people left in it. It is very unfortunate that so many of these good people have had their lives turned upside down.

I began my working career early by doing field work for local farmers. I was probably too young to do this kind of work but I wanted to earn my own paycheck. I got up at dark and entered wet, nasty, corn fields to detassle. For those of you who are unfamiliar to this, basically you would pull the flowery part out of the corn for pollination purposes. It was a dirty job we all hated but we did it to get spending money for the summer and upcoming school year. We started at day break, tromped through mud and cold wet corn leaves would hit you in the face and cut you. It seemed like the fields were ten miles long and we walked and walked. They have machines kids ride now but we didn't have them back then, it was all endurance and will. The afternoon would come and everything would dry out and get hot. It was like working in an oven with that sun beating down. Not a fun job but a job nonetheless. I hated the thought of it but did it every year I was in school regardless.

When I graduated High School I had to find a direction to head in. It is a pretty scary proposition to figure out what you want to do with your life. My idea of going into the military backfired and that was my big plan, to get money for school and not go in debt up to my eyeballs. It is hard to commit to pay 30 grand or more for college when you don't have a job or money. I decided to go to the community junior college and try to find a job from there. I graduated and worked many jobs, as I will touch on this later, but I ended up at a local factory. I was in my mid-twenties and it paid pretty well. It was a union job which appealed to me because my dad was union. I worked there as an operator and later went through an apprentice program to learn a skilled trade. After four years I became a journeyman millwright and really learned to like my job. The company I worked for treated me pretty good, I worked with a decent group of guys and life was going well. We were then bought out by a huge company with a lot to offer, and a lot of changes were made. They actually did their best to create a family atmosphere and a better work environment. If we had a gripe they would listen and actually attempt to rectify it. I remember when one of my co-workers had his house burn down right around Christmas. The whole plant took up a collection and the company matched what we had raised. The company bought presents for the family, helped him find another house, we handed him 13,000 dollars in cash. That is what I am talking about when you are proud to work for someone. You just don't see that kind of caring and generosity these days. It was funny because I would hear the chronic life haters talk about their job outside of the plant. But when people asked them if they liked who they were working for they would say hell yes, they treat us great. Something I haven't heard since they sold us.

Somehow this company got involved in the Enron scandal, I'm not sure what all happened but as soon as they had a bleak outlook they unloaded us. People didn't care about the reputation they just cared they were treated well and hated to see them go. We changed hands a few more times, went through a bankruptcy, as our President and his court made out with millions. And now we are run by a Texas outfit that has made life miserable. We have lost pensions, health benefits, and no pay raises for 5 years now. But of course the guys running the show are raking it in. It is an ethanol facility that produces bi products as well. I have been a union representative for the past ten years and it has been no picnic let me tell you. Every day is an unwanted fight and you are surrounded by unhappy workers. I understand it completely they have just been put through hell and are reacting.

All of those things my dad warned me about are coming to reality. He was just a dumb factory worker in the eyes of the golden spoon but a very smart man to me. He said there would be four dollar a gallon gas before Bush was through and he was correct. He said the price of gold and silver would skyrocket and once again he was right. He also warned pensions would be a thing of the past. Bingo. Dad was no prophet by any means but he was smart enough to see the writing on the wall. He had been seeing it for years before he died and I was amazed at just how smart that guy was later on. And all those things he fought for I understand now. The two tier wage system is the biggest scam in labor negotiating. Don't forget the dreaded signing bonus that you get half of after they rape you in taxes. There are just so many tactics he warned me about that companies would do to lower the standard of living it is scary. Now

I am living it. We are living it. It doesn't matter if you work in a factory or that superstore that keeps attacking wages, everyone is experiencing it. I'm just wondering how much the working man can take before things start happening. How soon before people get fed up? I think if you watch the news it is starting to happen. Not a very bright future for the kids is it.

The biggest fear of mine is the working conditions for people. My dad working in a foundry all those years died from lung disease. The cause of death on his death certificate was asbestosis, and believe me it is a long and painful demise. I can only hope in the years to come that someone will stand in and protect workers from the hazards they aren't even aware are killing them. My dad and his brothers all worked in factories except for 2 and only one of them survives. They all died in their forties, fifties, and sixties. And I told you of my grandpa earlier. I don't think it is coincidence by any means. Obviously it makes me wonder about my own span of life and if I will ever see retirement. I know retirement is a dirty word these days but I can hope can't I?

My parents both died horrible deaths and it pains me every single day when I think about it. My family doesn't even hear me discuss it because it is too tough to talk about. I am living with a wonderful girl I met about 8 years ago and her daughter that I have raised as my own. It is the only time they have seen my cry and I am not ashamed to admit it. It was the worst experience I have ever gone through by far and I don't wish it on anyone. My dad died from asbestosis as I previously stated, and my mom died from brain cancer 3 months apart from each other. It was a double header so to speak and not the kind I played in the back yard.

My mom was a good woman who stayed home with the kids while dad worked. We didn't have much and she was very frugal with what we did have. In the summer time we ate out of the garden that we put out, every meal it seemed. I like vegetables but everyone has their limit. We had corn, green beans, zucchini, tomatoes, squash, whatever we could pick. We also had cows that got out of the pasture once a week and we would have to chase them down. Hogs and chickens rounded out our barnyard extravaganza. So even though she was a house mom, that I think every family should have, she had her hands full every day. Handling us kids was no easy chore and it seemed like she was always in a good mood. Looking back I would have been in a bad mood all the time if I was her but she just took things in stride. She did what she had to do and was very organized. The house was always clean, the laundry was always done, I don't know how the heck she did it all but she did.

She was a very small woman under a 100 pounds all of her life, most people cannot believe I was a product of her loins. Her father was a very tall man, a skinny giant, and my grandma was a short woman but stout and tough. She grew up in a huge family by the local lake you can still see the frame of their house sticking out of the water when there is a summer drought. She really did have to walk uphill to school, not both ways, but she would show me the vacant lot where her little schoolhouse was. It was probably better than a mile hike, pretty impressive. So I could understand why we lived like we did. This is how she grew up and this is what she was used to. I appreciate it a little more now than I did then, as a kid seeing all the other things my friends had I didn't quite get it. I mean we had the things we needed, but little extra that other kids flaunted around. It really didn't bother me a whole lot, after all at one time we were all cramped in a four room house. Anything was better than that.

When I got in my late twenties my mom started having some problems with her kidneys. My grandma and grandpa had died from kidney cancer so this was nothing to play with. She being one not to gripe much started peeing blood and didn't tell anyone. My dad was already sick and she didn't want to be a burden in any way. Finally she went and got it checked out and the result was cancer in one of her kidneys. Eventually down the road they decided to remove her kidney. Everything seemed to go ok after a long recovery. She got back on her feet and was the same ol' mom in literally no time. She was fine for a couple of years and then the same symptoms came back, and our fears came back. She had a huge tumor that started where the kidney was removed and went to her liver. They said it was the size of a softball. We of course panicked and asked what we were supposed to do. In a nutshell they said nothing just sedate her and make her comfortable. The timeline was less than a year and it would be a bad year.

This is by far the worst feeling I have ever had hearing this kind of news. They said my dad was in final stages like 10 years ago and he was still getting around. We weren't going to give up but we had to convince her not to give up. She was the one going through everything, it was ultimately her decision. We finally talked her into going to Mayo Clinic in Rochester, Minnesota. They specialize in just about everything, what an amazing place with amazing people. There were 11 doctors from all over the world that looked at her case, each specializing in a different treatment for a specific body part. They collaborated and decided to try to remove the cancer. The doctors down here had the wrong type of cancer and were treating it totally wrong so thank god we got her out of there. We explained the sedate her and make her comfortable to die diagnosis and they laughed about it. They didn't accept mediocrity or failure, kind of what I talked about before. My dad was a nervous wreck and not doing well himself what a mess. But at least we knew mom was in better hands now. These were hands that cared about more than her checks.

Mom got ready to go to surgery and the doctors explained to us that it would be a long procedure. It would probably take 9 hours because the tumor was attached to her liver. This was not an in and out deal unless it was too far gone. If that were the case they would sew her back up and let nature take its ugly course. So if the surgery went quick it was a bad sign. Well after watching my dad freaking out which I had never seen before, the surgeon came out after an hour and a half. I remember dad saying oh no. To our surprise he said everything went great, they removed the tumor and part of her liver. She was now cancer free!!!!! You talk about a 100lb weight being lifted off your back I remember looking up to god and mumbling thank you. Our prayers were answered. What an outstanding institution Mayo Clinic was, I have nothing but good things to say about them.

We had to take mom back for a check-up every 6 months or so to make sure everything was still going well. She remained cancer free for 5 years, five years we were thankful to have. I sat down with her and talked to the doctors on one of her checkups. The cancer had reappeared and it was the size of a pencil lead. It was nothing to balk at but nothing to panic about either. They hesitate to open someone for fear of making it spread. We brought her back home and things seemed to be going normally. Then we noticed some changes in her behavior start to happen. She didn't talk much and she was starting to forget things. She hadn't fed the cat in a week which was unheard of, she absolutely spoiled that cat. The dishes sat for a long time in the dishwasher and she was washing them two or three times. My dad was starting to get worried as she complained of headaches which was never an issue before.

I remember the night like it was yesterday, my dad called and said something is definitely wrong with your mom. My sister and I went out to the house and she was a zombie. It was like she was really drunk. She was slurring her words and didn't make sense of anything she was saying so we took her to the emergency room immediately. She could hardly walk and it appeared she had a stroke, she kind of slid her feet instead of taking steps and she held her hand on the wall to steady herself. They did a scan on her brain and came back with the results. Cancer was covering her brain causing swelling which made her not function normally. My sister and I about dropped to our knees. I felt bad for my mom as she just kind of sat there smiling. I don't know how much registered with her but I am pretty sure she knew what was going on. The doctor suggested we take her back to Mayo and see if they could do anything for her.

We had to break the news to dad when we got home. They gave some medicine to mom to reduce the brain swelling which made a world of difference. She could now function normally and could speak intelligently. When I saw the life drop out of dad when we told him I knew it was over. He was going to give up his own fight from here on out. It took about 2 days and he was in the hospital. The game plan was I would stay down here in the hospital with him and my sister would take my mom to Mayo. My dad would hardly speak the entire time he was in the hospital but the one thing he did tell me was he was going to go before my mom. He couldn't stand to see her go through that kind of suffering and didn't want to be a burden on any of us. How do you handle this kind of situation?

My mom returned from Mayo and they were amazed at how well she functioned as bad as things were. They stopped at the hospital as she wanted to see my dad rather than go home and rest. She walked all the way up there and to the room. I was told the story before she went in that she would receive treatment down here because she didn't want to be stuck in a foreign place for weeks. I understood this and I knew she had to be home for dad. I walked in and told dad somebody was here to see him. Mind you these two argued all the time like the Costanzas on Seinfeld when they were together. They weren't happy unless they were bantering we noticed so we let them do it. My dad who hadn't spoken in a few days lit up like a Christmas tree. He reached up and smiled and hugged my mom like we were in a movie. To see a gruff guy like that sort of break down was pretty touching but in the same sense you get the feeling of how bad things really are. These two knew any time they had together was precious. And that was very sad to see your whole life come down to this defining moment.

My dad after this kind of sank back into his in and out state. I became very tired and finally went home to lie down as I hadn't really slept for days. As soon as I got home my sister called and said I better get back up there because dad was starting to swell up badly. My dad's twin brother died about 3 months prior to this and he did the same thing so I freaked. I got up there and my sister was right, his arms were about twice the size they should have been. I got ahold of his doctor and basically told him he needed to get his ass up there now! He finally showed up and went into his room and got dad to talk. This doctor had treated dad for years and my dad really liked him. They shot straight with each other on everything and had a pretty good relationship. He came out of the room and said you know he should have been dead ten years ago and he is tired. He is just giving up and I can't make him not want to give up. His kidneys are failing and we can do two things. If we get him started on dialysis right now we can save him. But your dad doesn't want that he is ready to go, it is up to you. There is nothing like a kick in the teeth with a life or death decision on your head. Dad heard us talking and said "hey get in here!" He basically ordered us to not put him on dialysis and to let him go, he was ready. I knew why and didn't argue with him. You can't take a man like that and make decisions for him it is his body, his mind, and his call. As much as it hurt there was no decision to make. No one knew how long it would be, hours, days, but he was going to die. And we let him have his dignity as he had all of his life. He was tired and ready to be with god and his family. How can you argue about that?

One part that made it also a little easier is that my father got things right with god recently. Not many people know but he had been speaking with a local pastor for a year or so prior to this. My mom was going to his church and took dad with her on occasion. He really liked the pastor and they became good friends. I was so thankful for that and it helped put my mind at ease about some things. We called him and told him to be by the phone because something was going to happen and most likely soon.

Mom went home to get a little rest the next day as they gave dad some morphine to make him comfortable. I on the other hand was not comfortable as my ears had plugged up. I could hear absolutely nothing. This was perfect timing, he could go at any time and I couldn't hear a thing. My brother took me over to prompt care to get my ears flushed out. I prayed he didn't go before I got back. Luckily they got it taken care of and I got back to the hospital before he passed. It wasn't a half hour and he began to writhe around. His blood pressure started to drop a little more at a time as I watched it like a hawk. I called my sister and told her to get my mom up there as fast as she could. He opened his eyes briefly and said get your mom frantically. I called them back and said HURRY. The pastor was already there so that was a good thing. My mom could only go so fast because she was terribly sick herself. Finally she made it and somehow he knew it. He was in a lot of pain and they gave him another shot of morphine, enough to put him in a comatose state. He started to get that death gurgle you hear about and his breath became shallow. It was coming and we knew it. He woke up briefly and said what he saw was beautiful. He started thrashing in the bed and somehow threw the covers off of him. His eyes were rolling into his head it was the most horrific thing I have ever seen. His blood pressure started dropping rapidly by 5 then by 10. The pastor did a prayer for him to introduce him to god. His entire family surrounding him watched him take his last breath. My dad and one of my best friends had died.

I looked up to the ceiling hoping to get a glimpse of him going to heaven and I remember hearing my sister screaming NO! Then I remember taking my hand off his lifeless hand and seeing all those years disappear in front of my eyes. That is all they were now, memories. Everyone was crying and I was angry at the world. A priest came up to talk to the family and I remember snapping at him of which I still regret to this day. I think I said something to the effect of you didn't even know him go away. It was strictly anger and hurt talking but I felt bad about it. I know that it was over now and he would want us to focus on my mom and get her through things.

My mom handled things well. The funeral and all that went as good as a funeral could go. I did have one melt down but I think I handled it like a man of which he would have wanted. My poor mom having to go through this knowing she was knocking on the door herself. What a strong woman she was, it was amazing. It was the hardest thing in our lives to go through and the worst pain to go through. I was so sick of being told I am sorry to hear about your loss. I know it is what you are trained to say in these uncomfortable situations but I just couldn't stomach it. I was jealous of people who had normalcy in their lives I was ashamed to say but it was just the way I felt and I had a hard time hiding it.

My mom wanted to be left alone I could tell but with her cancer we couldn't do that. We had to have someone there in case something happened. We also had to get through dads funeral bills, and get his stuff in order. It was a bad situation because we didn't have the opportunity to mourn. In addition we had to fight his insurance now that he was gone to cover mom in her upcoming battle. Our minds and bodies were trashed at this point. Even when you are at your lowest point things can never be easy can they?

We all tried to take turns staying with mom as she started radiation. My sister took a leave of absence from work and I tried to be there as much as I could while working. She didn't do too bad starting out but things started to go south quickly. Dad died in October and we were hoping to at least get one more Christmas with my mom. She began to get a horrible rash and started to lose her hair at a rapid pace. She began eating a lot and I mean a lot. The only thing we ever saw her eat were vegetables for the most part it was very odd. Her mind was still there and that was one of my biggest fears. It would be tough to deal with someone when they can't communicate what was wrong with them or where things hurt. I remember she called me at work one day all happy and told me my sister was letting her drive. It was nice to see her happy but in the same respect sad because this was such a highlight to her. A woman who did it all was so excited about driving around the block. I guess it gave her a degree of normalcy and a little control of her own. She could still do things other people take for granted. Mom hadn't felt in control or normal for a long time and she felt good about it.

We managed to make it to Christmas and it felt so weird with the way things were. It was the first one without my dad so we were all sad yet thankful at the same time. We knew it was our last one with mom and that weighed heavily on our minds. People were stopping by that never stopped by before and I know that made her feel uncomfortable. She knew that they thought she was going to die so they were coming to see her before it happened. I can't imagine how that would make someone feel. Of course no one says anything but you know when people are doing things they don't normally do it is because of urgency. We had an ok day but there was just so much out there to have a carefree time and enjoy it.

The days after Christmas things started to get bad rapidly, they wanted to put her on a new drug just introduced to the market and it had to be approved by insurance. It was like 500 dollars a pill. We needed it approved and approved NOW! The insurance denied it of course and we had to get documents from here and there. We went to dad's union president and he helped us get it through after a few blow ups. She started the medication and it made her very ill. She stopped eating and what little weight she had dropped rapidly. She laid in bed a majority of the time and was in great discomfort. Medication helped a little bit but she began to bind up inside. This caused excruciating pain for her, I felt so bad. Just imagine someone punching and kicking your mom and you are tied up with no way to stop it. That is what it felt like. We took her to the emergency room at the local hospital and after going through an hour of paperwork and a ten minute exam THEY SENT HER HOME. I was irate but she said just take me home. It was absolutely heartbreaking. By the time we got her home she was screaming in agony so we turned around and took her straight back. We didn't have time to get her to the better hospital in Peoria in this much pain. I got there first and let them know she was coming back. Do you know they made her go through all of the paperwork over again? This is no lie, the paperwork we just did that took an hour to go over we had to do it all over again. We were just there. I had a fit and threw a wheelchair off the wall. They urged me to settle down if we wanted her treated because this was standard procedure. I am sorry but when you see someone in that much agony standard procedure goes out the window.

After hours of waiting impatiently they finally got her comfortable and admitted. Mom was bound up and getting toxic because she couldn't get rid of her waste. This is the same thing that killed my uncle, my dad's twin brother. She had a high fever and was very sick. They tried an enema here and there but nothing worked. She woke up in the morning and there was a religious show on. They had the closed caption on the bottom of the screen. I remember mom spelling the words on the screen and pronouncing them. She said "see, I'm ok everything is ok"! She stayed awake a majority of the day and people came up all day long to see her. I think she stayed awake long enough just for that and then she started slipping away. It wasn't long after that her fever got worse and we were reliving what we just went through. We once again got the pastor up to the hospital and we all talked. Mom's blood pressure started to fall slowly. I began to hear that familiar gurgle. The entire family huddled around the bed, and I have a tear streaming down my face writing this. Her breaths were farther and farther apart. Then she just stopped breathing. Now my mom was with my dad. She was gone too. I once again let go of her hand and kissed her forehead. Life as I once knew it was over. My safety net was no longer with me, how will life go on from here?

When something like this happens you just feel empty. Like your tank is drained and you are somewhat angry. I had a nurse hand me a phone not five minutes after she died. I thought it might be a family member so I got my composure. It was somebody who was very sorry for my loss but wanted to know if I would donate my mom's eyes. Do you believe that? Five minutes after she died I kid you not. Do you have any idea how that made me feel? How insensitive could anyone be? I didn't blow up like my dad would have. I simply said they are not my eyes to give. And they were persistent, they would not take no for an answer. Finally I yelled NO and hung up the phone. And this time I didn't feel bad about being rude.

I talked to the doctor periodically during all of this but the statement that made the most sense came after she passed away. He said with all of the suffering she went through it was probably a blessing that she died. Sometimes the cure is worse than the disease. I thought about that and wondered if she would have had a better and longer life if we just let nature take its course. We all knew she was going to die but the drugs made her miserable and caused her death prematurely. I guess I will never know the answer to that question but I guarantee you I will think about that if it ever happens to me. There are a lot of lessons to be learned here.

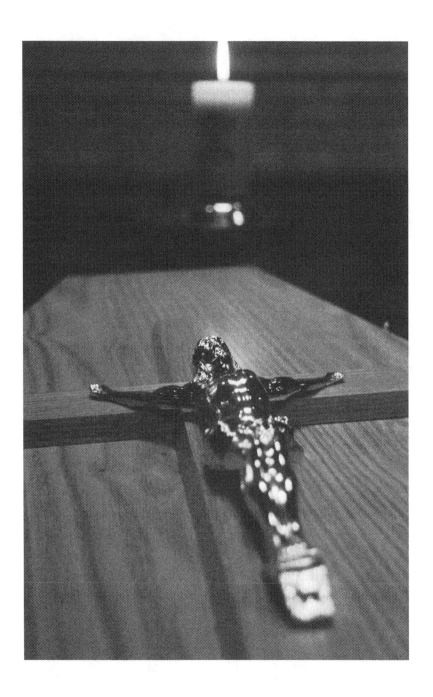

CHAPTER 6

After my mom's funeral I kind of became numb for a while and I kind of noticed that people really started to irritate me a lot easier. I would hear people whining about their petty problems and I would think to myself if you only had a clue. These people didn't know what problems were. My parents were both now dead and I was the executor of the will. I had so many things to do and not enough time to do them. My siblings and I went at one another's throats a few times as we all had different ideas on how to do things. I had medical bills coming in for the both of them that had to be paid and no one made it easy. I got double billed and triple billed for the same visit so I wasn't sure which bills were paid and weren't paid. We had a house full of stuff to go through and what to do with it. Man what a mess and what a job. I once again didn't have time to mourn and every visit I took to the house made me feel worse. I just wanted to crawl under a rock and die myself.

My dad went with me for lunch one day in famous Goofy Ridge about two months before all of this went down. We had liver and onions, and it was pretty good I remember it well. He was pretty sick and insisted on going so I obliged him. I don't know if he sensed it or what but he knew the end was near. He asked me if I would be the executor of their will. I asked if this would be the wisest decision because I was the youngest. One of my brothers lived out of state and the other wasn't around all that much. My sister would help me through it I was to hold the title. I didn't want to talk about this but he said "too bad" we are going to talk about it. I felt honored yet mortified because I didn't want to think about this stuff. It felt really weird. But I have to say I am so glad we did because I would have so many questions after they died. They had everything prepared for us. The headstone and the cemetery plots were already taken care of. Anything left after the funerals were over would be split four ways however we agreed to do it. I encourage you to have a talk with someone about these things just in case something might happen. It will make so much easier and there are so many things to consider.

You would not believe the amount of people that stopped by when we were going through stuff. Ironically my parents had borrowed so many things from people. If you knew them you would know that they never borrowed anything and if anything they gave away. A lot of these things I was with them when they bought them. But I thought to myself if you want it that damn bad take it. I had no strength to argue about it. Some people I had no problem giving some stuff to. I knew that they would have something to remember them by. And they waited for us to offer they didn't point at it and say it was theirs. It is amazing how greedy people get. I remember a quote from Planet of the Apes, "Man will kill his brother to possess his land." I don't think that quote was too far off base even though it wasn't his brothers. The premise of the statement says it all. People came out of the woodwork wanting this and that. We had to hide cars and not answer the door to get anything done and that is sad. And you knew what they wanted but they wouldn't come out and say it. They would lead into it and kind of slip it in there. They would tell stories of my parents and then relate it to the item that they wanted. It was really a work of art when you think about it.

My mom went through this when my grandma died and I don't think she would have been surprised. My dad would have cleaned house and been done with it. I remember my mom crying over the fact that as soon as my grandma's funeral was over the siblings started fighting over her things. Actually one my aunts didn't even come to my mom's funeral, her own sister's funeral for crying out loud. How sickening is that? All over money that happened 15 years ago. We were bound and determined this wasn't going to happen and it didn't thank heavens. But it took A LOT of patience. My advice is, have all of this in order because people will cut one another's throats over a wooden spoon. And that is the truth. Whether you want to believe it or not money is truly the root of all evil. I am speaking from experience here.

We basically had a drawing and did one room at a time. We would draw a number 1-4 since there were four of us. Number one would pick what they wanted and so on. It was fair and everyone got something that they really wanted. I would suggest this system for anyone going through this it makes it so much easier to deal with. The one thing I can tell you is don't get carried away because at first you want everything because it is so sentimental. I wanted that can of nails because we built the barn with them sort of thing. Then about four or five years down the road you ask yourself why in the hell do I have these nails? Just take the things you really want because after things die down you realize they are just objects. They are not the holy grail and a passage way to speak to the deceased. As insensitive as that is it is true. I have had others that have been through this say the same thing.

After we got everything divided up we took the rest to auction and received little or nothing for it. You think it is worth so much more because your mom and dad had it. I can assure you it does not work that way, it is the exact opposite. After we got that done we had to sell the house and what a pain in the ass that was. Selling the house was no fun. It was a beautiful place they took really good care of it, it was meticulous. Everyone that came through wanted this done or that done. No way either you want it or you don't. This had to be inspected that had to be inspected and someone had to be there when they did it. Someone finally bought it and drug us along for a month. We had the septic inspected and they said it was in great shape. These people wanted a new septic put in and got irate about it. We told them to eat it, once again either you want it or you don't. They ended up buying it and I drove by it a few days ago. It looks like a carnival in the middle of Old Macdonald's farm. It made me cringe but you have to let go.

It took about a year or so but I got everything paid for and enclosed the estate account. This was the most time consuming, mind boggling, experience I have ever endured. But when you take on a task your parents ask you to do it is your honor to do it. Plain and simple you just do it. I would like to think they are out there looking down and are proud of my family and the way we handled it. It is a tough ordeal to take on because everyone deals with death in their own way. Some want to be surrounded by people all the time and some want to be left alone. As a family you have to work together to be understanding of your siblings emotions and handle your own at the same time. This sounds easy but every time you pick up an object a new emotion goes through your head it never stops. We found out though if you have a good family foundation like we had, you know the one I have talked about that is ceasing to exist, you can get through anything. This doesn't mean you don't have arguments or you don't get mad because you will. In the end it is that bond you have built with your family with that stay at home mom that gets you back on track.

CHAPTER 7

Y ou know I have faith in god and he is my savior but I can't help
but wonder what happens when you exit this earth. I know there
is a heaven and it is a beautiful place, I have had two deaths door
testimonials on that. One of them, my dad, I already told you about.
The other one was my uncle that had multiple heart attacks within
a day. He died probably ten years or so before my dad. I remember
my dad kind of breaking down with this all going on. I won't go into
detail out of respect for him but let's just say I am the only one that
saw it. My uncle died a few times and they brought him back in
between heart attacks. Finally they decided to let him go or he just
couldn't take anymore. I never meddled to find out because that
was the family's business. He was a good man and we missed him
but I still have something that he wrote as he passed away. In case
you have any doubts this is what he managed to scribble covered in
tubes and in pain. As you will see it comes to an abrupt ending but
the message is clear. "When I was in the cather room (not sure) I
didn't know what it was until now but I saw the parts of Jesus that
everyone would like to see. He was the most shining and wonderful
person I have ever seen he has, and that is where it stopped. Now

when people write that kind of thing when they are just about to cross over it makes you think. At least it sure makes me think.

I have always had questions about what happens when you leave here. There are many interpretations but no one on earth really has the answers do they? For instance what body will I have in heaven? Will I be in a body at all? The one I died in at the age of whatever or the one I had when I was 18? I also wondered if people in heaven have any idea what is going on down here. Are they really around us all the time or just when we ask for them? To be honest I am human and it would be pretty embarrassing if they were indeed watching me all the time. I don't want them to see some of the stupid things I do on a daily basis. What if you were an infant when you passed? You really don't have thinking capability at that stage so are you a baby in heaven or are you grown up to the age you can function at? I know that your spirit leaves your body but that is a vague statement. Once again I have heard many interpretations of what is thought but no one knows. Let's say I love baseball here on earth is there baseball in heaven? Can I do the things I enjoy here up there or is it a whole different ballgame so to speak. Some would say yes and some would say no, it really isn't spelled out or at least I don't know about it. Will my mom and dad still be my mom and dad in heaven? Think about it how many generations of mom and dad's will be in heaven, how does that work? I thought maybe each immediate family would have their own little part but that would be complicated. Or maybe we don't remember any of it when we get there and are just happy that we are with god and in paradise. Some would say how could I question any of this? Well because I am human and god gave me a mind that tends to think from time to time. After all religion is a form of many different interpretations every church and every faction has their own beliefs. Catholics think way different than Baptist and I don't have the ability to say who is right and who is wrong. A bible verse can be presented in many ways and the interpreter has his or her own way of thinking. There would be a different answer for every question I have asked myself depending on where I looked. The bible is a fantastic compilation of teachings and stories to express the word of God and it leaves a lot of questions for us to figure out as any good book should. I plan on finding out the answers that is the important thing but I can't help but wonder while I am here on earth. I pray every night and try to live and do things the right way. I have met many people who go to church every Sunday and are the exact opposite of the person we are taught to be. They are greedy and rotten during the week and go church to be forgiven. I believe we are forgiven because it is written but I have a hard time believing that you can spend your entire life repeating this process. I can do something I know is wrong but that is all right because I will be forgiven no matter what. Maybe this is how it goes but it doesn't make sense to me and it isn't up for me to decide. I just try to avoid this way of living, limit my wrong doings, and try to be who God wants me to be. Of course I screw up because I am human but I try not to. There will be millions to tell me I am wrong for even questioning this but I have a mind for a reason and I like to use it. I am sure someone is pompously laughing out there because I know so little and they know so much that is how people are. I know I am not alone though as I have had conversations with people over the years and many ask the same questions.

In today's world when you turn on the television you basically have 4 options other than the religious channels if you have cable. You can watch war all the time, sports, reality smut, or some type of paranormal show. Whatever happened to Andy Griffith, (my favorite show), The Honeymooners, Gilligan's Island, and All in the Family.

All in the Family was considered on the edge at the time but it was a depiction of the way the world was then. Everyone I knew then was just like Archie Bunker, the world was Archie Bunker. What is wrong with telling the truth? It opened a lot of eyes. Bottom line is these shows were funny without cussing, taking off your clothes, or shooting someone. What is going to happen to television and the movies when they run out of things to talk about or the joke has been told so many times it isn't funny. I think we are getting to that point now. It is going to come down to the actor's ability to be funny with his character and not his script. People like Don Knotts, I don't know anyone that doesn't like that guys ability. The man was just funny. He didn't need to cuss or pull the trigger on someone to enjoy what he brought to the table. Now I have to admit Jackie Gleason did get raunchy but he was just as funny in The Honeymooners when he didn't. I did enjoy the Smokey and the Bandit movies I can't fib. I watch a lot of rated R movies but I am an adult and some of them are good. I'm not judging the one's making the money off it because it is reality of how the world is. I just think there is a place for it and a limit to it that's all. I think it is relied on a little too often these days on regular television instead of being naturally funny. I just wanted to throw my views on the tube out there. I know the older generation would tend to agree and the younger generation won't. But that is one of the few things we have left, a difference of opinion.

Since there is very little to watch on the screen these days I will from time to time check out the paranormal shows. Mind you, I try to have an open mind about everything but I like to have some kind of proof to substantiate it. Like I said earlier no one knows what is really floating around out there, and I don't persecute anyone trying to figure it out. But I guarantee you this, if I ever see an axe in the air, or a disgruntled moan telling me to get out. Guess what will happen?

You guessed it! I will heed that warning without a doubt. You will not see me in that location again, forever! I hear these people telling stories about waking up to a ghost sitting on the edge of their bed, or the apparition of a civil war veteran in their basement. And they continue to sleep in that bed, and continue to do laundry in that basement. Maybe I am a wussy, but I have news for you I AM OUTTA THERE! I don't care if I sleep in a barn I am gone. I am sure I am not alone in this way of thinking. And I listen to these EVP recordings with an open mind, most of them sound like garbled Alvin and the Chipmunks to me, all I hear is static. And if you convince yourself enough even static can sound like a word now and then if you want it to. I am not discounting it by any means but I haven't experienced it either. And there is always some sacrificial lamb that feels a tug or someone brushing up against them. Maybe in their mind they really do feel something, but at four in the morning in pitch black ghost like settings your mind is bound to play tricks. I think there is some validity to it but I also think it is stretched to make it entertaining.

Let's just say that some of this is true, and my view is there is no one out there that can prove that it isn't. They do come up with some pretty neat stuff and it makes you think if anything. Who are these spirits out there? Are they spirits that are damned or in purgatory? Are they the devil in disguise trying to convince us that there is no heaven? I remember one time when my dad briefly when in and out of life before he was saved. He spoke of this big valley full of people piled up on top of one another it was a dreary and gloomy place. The people were screaming to get out but had nowhere to go. This of course creeped me out to no end hearing this but was it reality? Something changed his way of thinking and it wasn't just mom getting on him. He saw something and did the right thing.

God gave him the chance and he was smart enough to take it. But where was this place? It was a far cry from the beautiful place he and my uncle saw before they died I will tell you that much. I often wonder was it purgatory or was it a glimpse of hell itself. Scary stuff either way and it leaves no doubt in my mind there are things going on beyond this universe. And it also makes me wonder if there are indeed souls out there that are lost and able to somehow communicate. Maybe they are there to send a message that this is what happens when you don't have faith? Maybe it is a big scam to capitalize financially on the unknown. Or maybe it is the ultimate unholy one creating a facade for the purpose of getting into open minds. No one ever admits to it but everyone thinks about it. Millions MUST think about it because it is flooding the television market more and more.

Another subject I try to keep an open mind about and a huge subject these days are alien life forms. I know it sounds crazy but I find it hard to believe that we are the only life form that exists in a huge galaxy. Isn't that kind of a pompous way to look at things? Just like dogs and cats exist here on earth that aren't considered human beings. No one really knows why they are here but they are, along with weird creatures like the squid, bugs, and birds. More advanced animals like the chimp and gorilla that have thinking capabilities like humans are among us. No one really knows why they are here and what purpose they have but they are even though we can't figure it out. Why would I be so self-centered to believe no other intelligent being could exist? I don't quite understand that way of thinking but I don't understand anyone's way of thinking these days. I am just looking at the basis of the subject, other life forms that can intelligently think. I have not made my mind up on spaceships and alien autopsies with Roswell and all of that. I know the government hides things this is what they do, but what do they gain by hiding a spaceship or a UFO sighting? And I am not saying that is out of the realm if there is some threat to humanity. I just am saying I myself have not seen any spaceships floating in the sky in my neck of the woods. In the same respect there are so many stories out there I am sure there are a handful out there that are legitimate. I mean you have military people and state police that have witnessed this kind of thing throughout history. These people have nothing to gain and everything to lose with their testimony. They are considered crazy from here on out, ridiculed, and die with no dignity. Even if they were paid would this be worth the price? This is what I personally look at when evaluating these claims but I have a unique way of looking at things.

I also have a hard time looking past the fact that these alien beings have been referred to since Egyptian times. I have always been taught to read the writing on the wall and they left it there for us to read. I find it hard to believe that they conjured up these images in their minds of spaceships hovering over the pyramids. And they would also be looked at as insane in those days. Egyptians had a heck of a lot more to lose back then being looked at as a nutcase. Image was everything during that period and I don't think someone was treated nicely as an outcast. So basically it took the entire civilization to be on the same page to create these images, even the leaders. It is hard to discount that many witnesses, including the civilizations half way across the globe who documented the same thing. There were no cell phones to communicate and these people documented the same things? How ironic.

And how did these pyramids get built anyway? They had no technology back then and the educated of today insist thousands of these little Egyptians hoisted these mammoth blocks precisely where they needed to be. I have been trained to rig heavy machinery and objects WITH modern technology and anyone who does this knows how bogus that theory is. It could not be done it just isn't plausible. I personally think they did have help in some way and they did have some advanced technology to assist them. I don't know who or what assisted them but you cannot convince me it was done the way laid out in the history books. But to me they gave us a clue with what they left behind even though we may never put the pieces of the puzzle together. There is something more to this.

And lastly my quest for the unknown leads me to this quest for Bigfoot, alias Sasquatch. I am sure you have caught a glimpse of this show at one time or another. Now this type of thinking totally makes everything I think about rational. It makes me differentiate life's mysteries from actual ignorance. I wasn't aware that we are now surrounded by colonies of sasquatches now shortened to squatches. These people also claim that there are skunk apes that live in alligator dens and forage for swamp apples. Of course there is no proof via picture or video to support these findings but they know they feed on bird seed, swamp apples, and candy bars if left out. They also know the blood curdling mating call of the squatch as they practice it and hurl it into the woods for response. Amazingly enough the squatch calls back and they KNOW it is indeed a squatch responding. It couldn't be some intoxicated guy a half a mile away doing a little night fishing could it? Now I know if you knew these people were going to be howling in the forest in your neighborhood you wouldn't mess with them. Would you? I would. But I know I have to be open minded they haven't proven they aren't out there. But this is the stupidest thing I have seen in a long time. I do get a good laugh out of it and I am hoping that was the intent. This is really taking advantage of our intelligence and satisfying the mentally challenged in the same breath. I am sure they have made a buck off it though because it is still on the air.

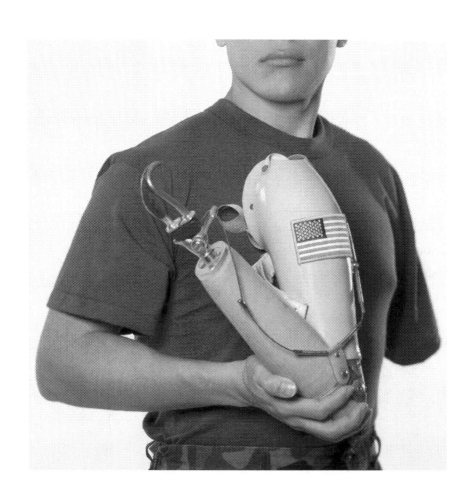

CHAPTER 8

Ironically today as I write this is the tenth anniversary of 9/11. It is of course plastered all over the television and it presents me with questions. What if this tragic event never happened? What would hold this country together? Thousands of people died and thousands still mourn it was a disgusting day in the history of our nation. I like everyone else is angry that it happened but I also look for the root cause. This is another one of those mysteries that I think we will never know as well. I know the story that is out there but I cannot help but think there is a little more to it. I just wonder what it really was that spurred these events and why these people had to lose their lives for it.

It is also disheartening that many blame this attack for the economic downturn of the United States. We saw a lot of people take the hit for it and we also saw a lot of people pad their pockets in between. It seems to me that anymore this is the only time that we see pride in this country to honor people that fall to senseless tragedy. I am watching the Chicago Bears today and I see probably the most gripping rendition of the Star Spangled Banner I have ever heard. The people were going crazy and waving the American flag and some had tears streaming down their faces. Once again you realize what makes this country what it is . . . . the people. They continue to get kicked in the teeth every day but they dust themselves off, get back up and wave that flag again. Isn't it sad that the only thing that we have to pull us together is the loss of life and being threatened? Why can't we be proud of other things, like the products we produce in this country? We could be proud that people are raising their kids in happy families living the American Dream. We could be proud that our government works together in pursuit of the happiness of the people that live here. We don't have to depend on foreign oil we could make our products here instead of Mexico and China. There are so many things that could pull this country together and make it great again but it will never happen. As long as the government can rely on the people pulling together when someone inflicts pain on us that is all they need. I am not condemning it by any means, I am proud of the people. But I know the government sits back and watches and says "see, there is nothing wrong here"! Tragedy gets them off the hook, it makes their job easier. Because they know we will watch out for each other and they don't have to.

Just look at how our disabled veterans get treated. These poor guys and gals risk everything they have including their lives to represent us. I can discuss this intelligently because I donate to the disabled veterans whenever I can. These people are forgotten in the government's eyes when they return with missing limbs or in a casket. These are the people that should be "bailed out". Instead you see the big ol' fat cats sending our jobs overseas whining and crying on their million or billionaire spreads. While the guy with no legs or the gal with no arms depends on people like me to help them get through life. I am more than happy to give what I can but these people should be put on pedestals and treated like royalty. And it should come from the government that sent them over in the first place. I know that when you sign on the dotted line you agree to battle but that also means there should be some responsibility for reward when you do your job. And this goes for the people lost in the twin towers, the surviving family, and anyone else involved. Take the golden spoon and start dishing some out to these people that lost everything for defending their country. There were billions of dollars out there given to those poor CEO's and these people live in poverty. What the hell is wrong with this picture? And the best reward is when they return to no job because it has been shipped overseas! How is that for a big thank you! And the people waving the flags are getting screwed just as bad, but everything is great isn't it? Remember my credit card story? Would there have been a story if a disabled veteran who needed a job answered the phone and talked to me? Or any other American who was currently out of work? I know it is just the way things are nowadays. I should smile and take it.

I also love it when people capitalize on other's misfortune even when they know it is dead wrong. How many people made money off of the "bloody glove" trial? If you murder someone and get away with it, hell you just won the lottery! You get million dollar interviews, a million dollar book deal this is quite a reward for allegedly killing someone isn't it? This guy was so confident in his status and fame he pushed the issue again with grand theft and finally got put away. Need I say more about the "Tot Mom" trial that just happened? How much money will exchange hands before that deal is over? She was an instant potential millionaire the minute she walked down those courthouse steps. A little girl is brutally murdered and people will profit from it. I just don't understand how anyone can seek reward for the death of a child. It is dirty money in my opinion but no one has a problem cashing the checks.

I guess I am the stupid one in the equation here because I haven't capitalized on how things are done. I tried to get in the military but I couldn't pass a hearing test. I wanted to defend my country and earn money for school. That is when it should have clicked. I should have researched sentences for certain crimes. Let us say I was caught selling cocaine and that was for the most part an eight year sentence. This would have been plenty of time for me to get my master's degree in just about anything I wanted. I would have plenty of study time, free room and board, meals, and best of all a free education that you paid for! No student loans, no bills, no working while studying, no headaches. When I got out I could find a job because I was rehabilitated and someone could make money taking a chance on an ex con. I would be in my mid-twenties, with a master's degree and my whole life ahead of me. But I didn't. I did things the right way and struggle like most of the people reading this.

Now I know there are a lot of prisoners out there that want to strangle me because they are in there and I am out here. I don't know what it is like and don't want to know for that matter. I just am frustrated that people get rewarded with opportunity for being bad, and people get punished for being upstanding members of society. Surely anyone can understand that way of thinking. And I also know there are a lot of innocent people behind bars as we speak. Some people are put there because our judicial system is a joke. People who murder get out in under 10 years sometimes and others for less offenses stay in for life. And sometimes people get incarcerated just because they are the most logical person they can find and don't have millions to defend themselves.

I have a cousin that is currently serving two consecutive 99 year sentences for alleged child molestation. I will never understand that consecutive sentence thing when no one has lived to the age of 198.

This mind you is without the possibility of parole. I don't know my cousin all that well and I don't know if he did it or he didn't do it. But here is the story I heard from behind the scenes. He decided to play around with another friend's wife. I know this a bad thing but no crime in the court of law. The disgruntled husband found about it and vowed he would get revenge. I went to school with this guy and he is a shady person, and that is putting it nicely. I have no doubt in my mind that this could have been the case, it happens every day. I was not in the courtroom but all indications point that the kids he allegedly molested were told what to say and the stories varied every hour. These were the revenge seeking husband's kids in case you have not guessed. What better way to get back at someone who had a fling with your wife than send them to jail for life? My cousin is a poor man who could not afford a lawyer so you can imagine the representation he received. The judge promptly made an example out of him and put him away forever. This is fact as he sits in prison as we speak waiting to die.

Now we talk in this country about the ability to rehabilitate and make people active members of society. We spend an ungodly amount of money doing it. To me even if he did this, which is very suspect at best, isn't this the type of behavior that could be rehabilitated? I'm sure 10 years in that hole could convince anyone that this was a bad choice on its own. You see murderers on the street, you see people on death row released. But this is the sentence that warrants 198 years in prison? If he did do it he should pay for it and pay for it dearly, but with his life? And no one really knows if he did it in the first place, due to the circumstances probably not. Castrate the guy if you have to but I can't see locking him up until his funeral. I had 2 convicted sex offenders on my street that served 2 years or less, guilty or not guilty. I always wonder if some type of dispute put them there or they really did it. If my dad told me what to say, you are damn right I would say it. He would never do that but I know there are people out there that would coax their kids into lying. There are parents who would take advantage of their child's vulnerability and brainwash for their own benefit. People kill their kids for their own benefit for crying out loud. It is sickening what some will do. It is just insane how horribly the court system works for the money we spend on it. If you have a repeat offender with a prior record that is a different story and not what I am referring to, they need to be dealt with. To me there are just too many question marks out there these days and too many people who play the courts like a fiddle to be sure someone is guilty. It is also too easy to put someone away because they lack the money to defend themselves. If you have money you can get out of it we see it time and time again. If you don't and you really aren't guilty you are screwed. Child molestation is a sick and disgusting act but the court system has made it a sure fire way to put someone away without concrete evidence unless you have a wad of cash. If there is evidence other than hearsay put them away but there are a lot of people behind bars that didn't do it. There are so many people using this as a way to get even and that isn't what the courts are about. There are a lot of cases where the children later admit they were coaxed to lie or their words were taken out of text and this shouldn't happen. It is a fine line I know and I sound like an advocator of molestation, no way. I'm just saying it should take more than hearsay to convict just like in murder trials. If hearsay was enough we wouldn't have many politicians left in office would we? Our children should be protected and cherished but we also have to realize they are taught what to think and to say. Most kids have a limited thinking capacity and some parents would take advantage of it for their own motives. This is sad but it is the world we live in.

I mentioned the disabled veterans earlier and that is a donation I try to make on a regular basis when I can afford it. Another donation I try to give to is St. Jude every year. Everybody has their hand out these days because our government who loves us can't seem to distinguish the difference between need and greed. We have sick children out there dying every hour and suffering every minute. Yet we flip the bill for private planes, lavish dinners, vacations among other things. We need to make sure our CEO's and members of political parties have these things, it is vital they don't do without. And there lies a little sick kid in a hospital bed and their parents in disbelief. They don't know where their next meal is coming from on top of the stress of a suffering child. We as a society dig in to our pockets to make a dent in the despair and try to help in some way. These huge companies that we bail out and move our jobs overseas give a token to say they are a company that cares. But who do they take it from? It certainly doesn't come out of their pockets. It comes in the form of wages and benefit packages from their employees. It comes from the pensions they take away and retiree health care they abolish. It comes from moving the jobs to Mexico and China so they can get by cheap. Who still ends up taking care of their own? That's right, the true American waving his flag at the Bears game. I know that a lot of sports figures put back into society and help sick children. Kudos to those individuals but it isn't enough. These people that go through this sort of thing should never have to worry about a light bill or a car payment. They should be able to focus on what is important, the life of their child. Wouldn't some of the billions we waste frivolously on the upper crust be more suited to take care of our sick and make some lives a little better? I know that's just the way it is these days. How uneducated of me to think in those terms.

I am in no way shape or form knocking educated people. It takes sacrifice, work and money to become educated. Our country needs to be more educated I keep hearing. What I don't hear is who is going to pay for it. How can the lower middle class afford to send their kid to college? Every dime they make goes to increased health care and the cost of EVERYTHING! Basically it goes like this, they spend 60k to 100k for school themselves to make 35k to 60k or a little more if they are lucky. The price of everything doubles or triples by the time they have their own kids ready to go to college. Now they can't afford to send their kids to get a higher education with the rising cost. They do it anyway because they want their kids to have a chance. The price of school goes up every year, they spend their savings and retirement, and their kids are making less money than the parents are when they graduate. That is if they find a job in the first place! The parents are not only still paying for their own student loans they are paying for their kids too because the kids aren't making enough to pay it. If you are really lucky and your kid is an athlete, they can get a free ride! Even if he or she is as smart as a thumbtack it doesn't matter. I am a sports fanatic and I watch college sports religiously. But this is absolutely ridiculous to discriminate against someone because they can't dribble a basketball or hit a 400ft. homerun. There are grants out there for the non-athlete but they don't touch the costs that go into four or more years of school. But the defining factor that is never addressed is this. All people have a different level of intelligence. Not everyone can be a college student it just isn't in the cards for them. As hard as they try they just aren't blessed with that kind of capability. Translated by the upper class it means they are insignificant and no longer useful. They should be treated as such and receive none of the things that contribute to a well-rounded American family. If you cannot achieve a piece of paper with the word degree on it you are now considered dirt. Peasant would be the word I am looking for. And it now has extended to people who are by definition educated but not educated enough. It has turned into a free for all no one is safe except for the boys at the top and their supporters in government. The most educated people on the planet are making decisions about your life and how you live it look how that turned out!

I agree that with hard work comes reward but who defines hard work? I believe that the person who makes the golden spoon should be rewarded as well as the person who eats from it. After all if no one MADE the golden spoon no one would be EATING from it now would they? People who work their way to the top should be paid for it. WITHIN LIMITS!! The people at the bottom should be able to enjoy life too but fact of the matter is they can't. This is not in reference to those people who refuse to work and abuse the system. This is not in reference to people who buy a 200 thousand dollar house, can only afford a 60 thousand dollar house and expect to be bailed out. I am referring to the single mother who makes 9 dollars an hour and spends 10 dollars an hour for day care. I am referring to two working parents that can't afford to take their kids to a ball game or a movie. The people who keep the country running need to have enjoyment too! Isn't that what life is all about?

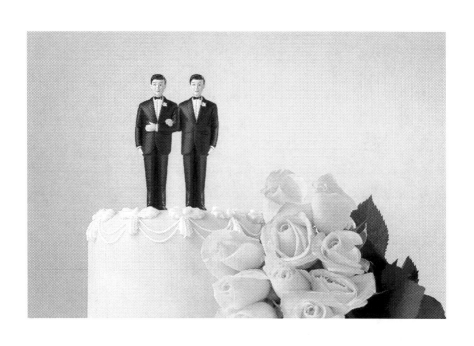

CHAPTER 9

Every day is a constant reminder of how the world is changing at a rapid pace. I don't see how anyone can keep up. It seems like we focus on the most insignificant things while it all just crumbles around us. What is the deal with our continuing focus on gay marriage? Is this really a significant issue with things the way they are right now or political positioning. Come on do I really care if two gay guys or two lesbians get married? No. But I do have a problem with it getting special attention and special rules. Does it have to be flaunted? What two people do behind closed doors is none of my business or concern more power to them. But I also don't feel we need to have lavish mardi gras like parades and force people to be a party to it. What kind of a stir would I raise if I had the straight man parade? This would be considered a waste of time and it should be. Why would I promote it? I consider this in the same capacity of a gay parade, no reason for it other than try to cram it down my throat and flaunt it.

When I was a kid we were good friends with a family that had a gay man in it, a brother of the family. I know it drove my dad crazy but he kept his cool about it. This was just not accepted in his generation. No one persecuted him or made him feel unwanted but this guy continued to make it uncomfortable and push it on people. I remember when some guys came to fix some lines outside of their house one summer while we were visiting. Most people would just let them do their job and leave them alone. This guy puts on a tube top grabs his paton and starts twirling it in the yard in front of these workers to woo them. This is no lie I remember it like it was yesterday. The workers didn't say anything but the looks on their faces said it all. They are screwed because if they say anything they are gay bashers so they did the right thing, their work. But what gives this guy the right to make these guys feel uncomfortable and embarrass them? Would this be considered sexual harassment on the workers part if they said something or considered violating his gay rights if he wasn't allowed to EXPRESS himself? I highly doubt the workers would have a leg to stand on. That is what I mean about special treatment. I don't broadcast to the world I am a straight man nor should they broadcast to the world they are not. I don't care if they get married but pay the taxes. I don't care if I work with a gay or lesbian just don't expect special treatment from me because of it. I mentioned earlier that I didn't get into the military because I could not hear well enough to pass the test. If I were gay and didn't get in would have a million dollar lawsuit regardless of the reason? I believe no one has a choice if they are gay or straight and it is no one's fault for whatever reason people are born this way. And I don't think people should be discriminated against because of it. I say equal rights but that means EQUAL RIGHTS. I can see in the future that a company will have to hire a gay or lesbian to fill a quota and that is just dead wrong. If they fit the job and are qualified fine but no special attention should be given for ones sexuality just as it shouldn't be discriminated against. I think some only want that, but from what I see and hear many want more, a lot more. I am not willing to give it, sorry.

When I go to the voting booth I believe there are a lot more important things to address like the ability for people to have affordable health care and take care of their kids. I know people vote solely on the abortion issue, gay rights, among other things. I am not disregarding the importance of these issues but don't we have some bigger fish to fry at this point? However anyone votes is their business but first things first, get the country back in business and go from there. We have spent so much time as a country focusing on "other" things our backbone has disintegrated. It is time to prioritize because if we don't act swiftly it will be too late. It may be too late already.

It seems like I am supposed to give accolades because someone comes out of the closet. Let's say a prominent sports figure announces to the world that he is gay or she is a lesbian. Quite frankly I don't care. If they hit 40 home runs I will remember them if they are gay or not, if they win Wimbledon was it because they are gay? No, they are a good tennis player. I heard someone say something about a certain general manager in the major leagues. Isn't he brave for telling people? Imagine that, a gay man in the major leagues, what an icon. What bearing does being gay have on anything? Why should it? He is a good general manager that is all that matters. I know there are many straight general managers in the major leagues, are they icons because they are straight? Please explain it to me I don't get it. Treated equal or treated special? I know it is a touchy issue but many people feel the same way and it should be said. Like it or not.

Where I come from I will be ridiculed for even implying equal rights but that is how I see it from my point of view. There are so many people left out there that won't even budge on this issue and would cure it with a baseball bat. That is just the way society is in the rural community and that is wrong. But perhaps if things were portrayed a little more tactfully and a little less flamboyantly things might get done. Like I said the day in and day out media coverage of gay parades really kills any movement of this issue. I am watching late night television and notice the gay and lesbian comedy hour and once again didn't see the listing for the straight comedy hour. Some of it was kind of funny but some of it was kind of overboard too. I thought to myself some of the people I know would kick the television in if this came up. I think the flamboyancy of the whole thing turns people off and limits their ability to be open minded. Rather than the LOOK AT ME I AM GAY approach, how about the yeah I'm gay but I am just like you approach. Agree with me or not it is how people think and there are millions shaking their heads yes while reading this. A little normalcy added to the equation would go a long way.

I entered the redneck fishing tournament in Bath, Illinois a few months ago. And yes that is exactly what it was, REDNECK. In case you don't know what this is, it has become a national event televised on the Travel Channel, ESPN, National Geographic, to mention a few. The Asian carp epidemic has been an ongoing concern in our river system and continues to get worse. They continue to rapidly multiply and eat the food sources of other fish, they are a garbage fish. They are not an edible fish and are eating machines. When you take a cruise down the river you will see these fish jump behind the boat in huge numbers. Commercial fishermen have been put out of business as they are trying to find ways to harvest them usefully. Bath residents decided to do their part to get rid of them in their own way. Basically they have a contest once a year and people go out with their dip nets, baseball bats, and try to fill their boats. The boats huddle together and the waves created provoke the fish to jump, you then try to get them in the boat any way you can. They have several heats and whoever has the most fish per heat in their vessel wins a cash prize. My brother, nephew, brother in law, and I entered into this not really knowing what we were in for. It was the most chaotic, nerve racking thing I have ever been involved in. There would be ten or more boats all within a couple feet of each other. It was just like the part in jaws when they all go out of the harbor to get the shark, man it was freaky. These fish that get very large would be flying by your head smacking people in the face. Needless to say we didn't win but we lived through it and that was a victory in itself.

Bath is a very small river town in Central Illinois, and the clientele is unusual to put it mildly. They are very friendly people but it is obvious the lack of a dental plan that exists in this area. They drink a lot and swear even more but I was amazed that there wasn't a lick of trouble. There were thousands of people I would guess and nothing got out of hand. They just had a good time and did ask my family to show their breasts on occasion but meant no harm. They had a costume prize as well. I was graced by the presence of the Easter Bunny, the Beatles, Hulk Hogan, Vikings, all kinds of famous people. It was pretty fun I have to admit I had a good time too.

These were good down home people but not what I would consider advocates of the gay and lesbian communities in other parts of the country. I wondered if someone paraded around this type of atmosphere with a sign stating they were gay what would happen. I think I know the answer to that question and it wouldn't be good. This would not be perceived in a positive way. Most likely someone would have gotten hurt and there would have been trouble, big trouble. But what if that same someone just had a beer with a few people and wasn't flamboyant about it? If they had the opportunity to know the person a little and saw they were just there to have fun like everyone else? The outcome would be way different I guarantee.

People don't like things forced on them, especially when they don't believe in it. And whether gay or lesbian people like it or not there are millions of down home people out there and that doesn't mean they are bad people. Maybe they don't believe in what you do, so what. This doesn't mean they won't let you live among them, they just don't want to live it themselves, or be forced to believe in it. That is their right too. Or should I say equal right. Gay bashing is totally stupid and I don't condone it, but there has got to be a better way to fight it. No matter how you slice it there will always be violent, ignorant people out there. But as a whole people are not and respond in a positive way if approached in a positive way. That is all I am trying to convey here, something to think about, something I hear every time the subject is brought up around me. Sometimes the voice of the average person living life makes a little more sense. Rather than an egghead telling how people are supposed to feel about it or they think this way because they were spanked as a child. This is reality.

We live in a society where we like to talk about issues but we can't say this word or say that because it might offend someone. These days no matter what you say someone is going to be offended that is what we have created. Even though it isn't right life isn't always nice to us. I am fat if someone calls me that they have just stated the obvious. I AM FAT! Do I need to launch a parade for overweight people like myself, or sue the individual that called me this? It is my own fault that I have become fat no one else. If it is genetic, it still isn't their fault. Just the card I was dealt. I am accountable for what I put in my body I am not blaming anyone else. This is how I feel about it. I know I am not supposed to eat it, I know the end result, but I do it anyway. Obviously I don't love being called fat and I WILL RESPOND in some way, but to blame it on the person who says it as the cause, baloney. I'm not fat because I was spanked as a child for being disruptive. I am this way because I eat too much and exercise too little. I don't need a pity party and a support group, I need to motivate myself. I know people have self-esteem or underlying issues and need help. Sure people need a kick in the butt sometimes and after they lose the weight I think they realize it was laziness for the most part or lack of knowledge of how to do it.

Look at how many people profit by convincing us it isn't our fault. The catch phrase is "Diet and exercise don't work, we understand it's not your fault." Then they promptly charge your credit card as show of concern, with the little caption on the bottom, results will vary with DIET and EXERCISE! People make billions taking advantage of your vulnerability with transparent notions of caring how you feel. If they really cared how you feel they would send it for free wouldn't they? I don't think so. Psychologists will gladly take a 100 dollars and hour to convince you the things you have done aren't your fault. My dad swatted me for being an ass so everything I have done is his fault. What are we doing here? We are paying people big money for them to shift the blame to make us feel better. And they are right there to take it. I could write an entire book on the ignorance I have displayed over the years. And there are people out there reading this that will surely support this claim. I have gone insane on several occasions and pulled some idiotic stunts. I look back and ask why I did it and still have no idea. We have all done this we are human beings. People in government do the wrong things every day. Our beloved CEO's screwing everyone and laughing all the way to the bank. But it is just how the system works, if they could do something they would, it's not them. It is never anyone's fault is it? We have created a society where no one is to blame for anything. All we can do is do our best and accept what we have created individually, move forward, and hope morality will play a part someday.

I have stated earlier my firm belief in Christianity, and I also believe that god doesn't care about money. You see it every year some evangelist gets popped for stealing money. I understand that a church needs money to function and a pastor or minister has to eat too. This is not an issue to me in the least. Spreading the word of god is a full time job and everyone should make a living. I am writing this book to spread the word of a common man and maybe make a living too. I cannot cast stones for that. My question is, how do these big money evangelists get away with it as long as they do? Isn't better to give than to receive? Trust me I live by this and why I have nothing and others will attest to that. They have these huge gold rings on their fingers, necklaces, 1000 dollar suits. They broadcast from these million dollar castles and sit on gold thrones like kings when they give the message. Why wouldn't anyone who truly believes in god question this? They are telling me I need to send my paycheck to help the starving in other countries. God will reward you for this, if they get it. Do these people honestly think the messenger is sending HIS PAYCHECK? Come on man they have more money in the watches on their wrists than I have in the bank. These are intelligent people sending everything they have and entrusting it in these hands. The list is huge of people that have stolen millions some convicted some not. The people who have been stolen FROM continue to stick up for them. These con artists take advantage of that word again, vulnerability, of honest people trying to do the right thing. No person would ever use God as way to get rich. You bet they would and they do it every day of the week. It has been going on for years, the Jim Jones tragedy I would have thought would open some eyes, but it got worse after that! They pay big money to hear someone say, "it is not your fault, god will forgive you" people will send money for this message. God WILL forgive you! But not because you send these convicts a check every week. It is god's work to give and you can't fault anyone for that. I just can't understand why people can't see where it is going when it is right in front of their eyes.

I know it is a pretty sad state of affairs when the place we go for worship, peace, and tranquility, are a melting pot of greed. Unfortunately greed has no boundary it will get you at the grocery store, mailbox, and even church in some cases. There are millions of upstanding churches out there and I commend every one of them. You generally only hear about a church when something bad happens I realize because good doesn't sell like it used to. I just hope people wise up and start putting these millionaires out of the picture. I am sure the penalty will be much worse later on down the road when the ultimate judge gets ahold of their portfolio's and renders a verdict. But it would be nice to save a few lives of others in the meantime wouldn't it?

The worst part is that the people that get taken advantage of the most are the people that should be cherished, our senior citizens. This in itself tells you what the country is as opposed to where it was. These people lived in a day and age where people trusted one another. They could donate money and it actually went where it was supposed to. I just wonder how they can just not sit and look at a wall in disgust of the way things have become. People go door to door telling them they need this and need that, steal everything they have and move on to the next. Their retirements get squandered in some Ponzi scheme and they get conned into these reverse mortgages. The very people we are supposed to take care of the most are the ones that get pounded the hardest. It just isn't right. No one protects them they just make it more difficult to get through each day. Can you imagine trying to live in the world today as a senior and survive with the way technology changes? That would be one scary deal and they get taken on things as simple as an oil change or painting the garage on top of it. You know if an air conditioner goes out in an elderly woman's home she will end up with a new unit she can't afford. The scariest part is we live in a society where people could care less. My grandma used to walk to the store and the post office when I was a kid to get exercise. My mom of course offered to take her but she liked to get out so she did it on her own. I would be scared to death to see her do that now. Kids would take her purse or throw rocks at her, call her names. Gangs steal from them, invade their homes, and even rape them in some cases. It must be horrible living your golden years in that type of world and no one to help you. They of course get rewarded by getting less money to live on or put in a home with sub-par living conditions if they don't have the cash. It just breaks my heart to see people that gave us the opportunities we have get treated with such disrespect. I would give everything I have to get my parents and grandparents back but part of me is thankful they don't have to live through this. I can't fathom what it will be like if I make it to that age. Of course all those upper crust people have it covered, champagne and cruises. I just tend to worry about those that don't have those luxuries. I know that is just the way it is. I should focus on the important political issues like gay and lesbian marriage.

I always got made fun of because I would get on anyone and everyone for littering. I would lay out a vision of me in my golden years sitting on the porch in my rocking chair trying to rock through the garbage. Little did I know then I wouldn't be able to afford a porch or a rocking chair. My friends would throw something out the window and look over and see me glaring. They could recite my rocking chair story word for word. It was funny and we would chuckle about it but I was serious. Man are we destroying this land that we live in. That is one thing I will say this country is trying to put a little more emphasis on pollution and going green. People get made fun of and called tree huggers in these parts but damn somebody is going to have to start taking care of things. I remember stories of my dad and grandpa (mom's dad) talking about the river being crystal clear and being able to see the bottom ten feet out. Other people have corroborated these stories as well. It is so polluted now it would gag a maggot, yet no one cares. Just how things are these days I have been told. How long does the world think mother nature is going to put up with this? I am looking out the window now and seeing garbage in the neighbor's yard, it bugs the hell out of me. Not only do we have to find a way for it to not pile up on the streets we have to find a way to contain it. Just think about how much garbage you and your family produce a week on your own. How about a year? Where the hell is all this garbage going? It goes to landfills and into the ground if it doesn't get into the water or dumped somewhere. How long can we continue to do this before it bites us? It is contaminating our water as we speak and I don't see it getting any better. I have a grand kid on the way and I would like to have a world for him or her that enables them to get a drink of water without getting sick. This doesn't even scratch the surface of what big industry is doing to the environment. Big oil has done wonders in the past few years haven't they? I know we don't have to worry it isn't about money, our big industry and government will do whatever it takes to make us safe where we live. I see commercials about it every day, not to worry, we are a great nation! I have news for you I am worried about it and everyone else had better start worrying too if you have a kid in the mix.

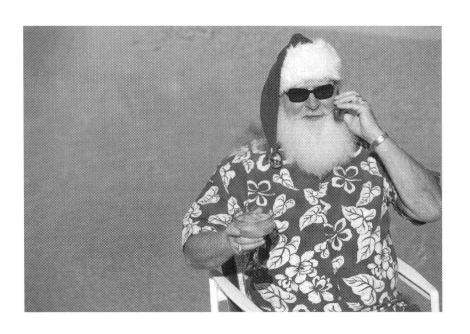

CHAPTER 10

One of the other things that keep our American families glued together would be the holidays. I have learned in addition to god needing money, Santa Claus also needs money. What a money making enterprise in good old Saint Nick. Evidently the North Pole has become a pretty pricey venture these days. The elves must have unionized and started putting a dent in Santa's bottom line. Does Santa have a health care plan and retirement for those hard working elves? Perhaps he should think about moving his operation to a warmer cost saving climate such as China or Mexico. I am sure if our leaders sat down with him they could show him how he could have China or Mexico save him a boatload of money. They could make the toys for below poverty wages, pay no benefits, no vacation time, no sick days, what more could Santa Claus ask for? Free labor and he could even outsource his reindeer to save another buck. He could use camels to deliver the toys to all the boys and girls! As stupid as that sounds do you think if Santa Claus were real this wouldn't be happening? He would have a board of directors raking in millions and the little elves would be in cages eating straw to survive. And everyone would say that's just the way it is these days. Those elves should be happy they have a job.

Seriously, doesn't it bother anyone that this sacred holiday has become this money making cut throat industry? Christmas used to be a time to celebrate the birth of our lord and savior Jesus Christ. It has now turned into a holiday to celebrate 30 percent off at Target. I know it is a season of giving which is fine but to what extreme? I believe I received NOTHING from my employer but the CEO received a 7 million dollar bonus. That is the holiday spirit isn't it? When I was a kid I remember getting one thing for Christmas maybe two. The cool part was I was happier than a pig in shit to get that. These were cheap items as well, I have a picture with my brother holding a basketball, other brother had a GI Joe, sister got a Miss Beasley doll, and I got a Winnie the Pooh. That was it and we were thrilled. We even took a picture to record the smiling faces. How much do you think the average family spends on Christmas now? I am sure there is some statistic for it but I would say at least 500 dollars on the low end. And I know there will be many that argue that is way too low. What the hell happened to distort this most sacred of all holidays? I have two words for you corporate greed!

Corporations feed and prey on that big money making word . . . . vulnerability. After all we have the technology to expose this in every way. The television is plastered from October on with what all the other kids are getting for Christmas. If your kids don't get it you are a worthless and your kids considered neglected because of this. Every parent wants the best for their kids and how do they feel if little Johnny gets a Red Ryder bb gun and the annoying snot nosed brat down the street gets a high powered rifle? It makes them look inferior, embarrassed, and it is perceived they don't care about their kid. As selfish and disgusting as that is that is how our society works. Everything is based on perception of what others think. I am just as guilty of this and I am trying to change it. I just saw an ad today of how every kid needs a smartphone. Can every family afford to get their kids a smart phone? Absolutely not, but they will do it because the ad tells them they have to have one to be smart. They make you feel vulnerable and guilty if every kid has one but yours. Your kid has to have it to keep up with the other kids in today's technology. If they don't they will fall behind and be considered an idiot by societies standards. A parent cannot win in any situation and people have the audacity to ask why families live beyond their means. They don't have a choice, they are perceived as people who don't care about their kids and keeping up, they are cheap, or go in debt and can't pay their bills. The golden boys laugh and laugh all the way to the million dollar club. Makes you proud doesn't it?

My parents never let me forget the true meaning of the word Christmas and what it was about. It was simple, being with family and celebrating the birth of Christ. Gifts were third priority if not lower on the list. Corporate America has even ruined that haven't they? Usually in most families one of the parent's has to work on that day to pay for thousands they forked out to make little Johnny and the economy happy. I would say in ten years there will be very few paid holidays left except for federal holidays that our members of government have to have. You wouldn't expect them to be like us of course. The higher paying jobs would retain theirs because of all the stress they go through during the year. None of us have that to worry about. We should be happy to work on a holiday to get those hours and be happy to have a job! Family doesn't matter we get at least 10 hours a week with them. Some people will read this and laugh but this is REALITY and most of you can relate to it.

What do you think is going thru the mind of god when he sees the main event, Black Friday? At least they got the name right on this one. This is where people camp out in frigid weather to get that deal they can't afford. There is usually some kind of altercation as people get irritated with each other waiting and waiting. It is a season of giving and usually someone gives a punch in the face as a present. Corporate America sits on their golden throne filling their fat guts and giggling at our stupidity. They sit back and anticipate this year's bonus while the masses become restless and frostbit. We are at their mercy and will risk injury and death to get a crumb from them. It is even on play by play as every news outfit is there to broadcast our great nation in their proudest of moments. Finally after 12 hours the doors open and the cattle begin herding and then erupt. People get trampled, punched, beaten, verbally assaulted, or killed. Most come out empty handed but some come out with the mother load and have spent ten times more than they anticipated. Exactly what the big boys hope for. And people do this why? So they don't feel guilty that little Johnny didn't get what we were told he had to have. And most spend the rest of the year and or the rest of their lives paying off the credit cards that are already used to pay the light bill. This is a vicious cycle that has become a Christmas tradition in this great country of ours. By the way, Happy Birthday Jesus!

You have noticed I used the term Christmas on several occasions. We are now told that Christmas is a bad word, the term holiday is more politically correct. Well guess what? I refuse to conform to these rule changes and have two words for anyone who disputes it. Quite simply, bite me! I really could care less what any other culture might celebrate I live in the American culture that was created by Americans for America. I think celebrating what people believe in is great. Just don't expect me to change what I believe in and what I celebrate in MY country. I admit I get a little frosted at society and the new generation but the goal is to restore what made this country great in the past. CHRISTMAS is a part of that and I will not give that up. Despite the brainwashing techniques of the people that devise these things through the media, I have a few million people to back me on this one I guarantee. You may have destroyed the concept of Santa Claus but when you tread on the heels of our lord's birth, you are going to get a fight. Leave it alone!

CHAPTER 11

Throughout this book I have referred to technology on many of occasion. I have been trying to re-enter the workforce in a different capacity. I have worked in a factory for a majority of my life and I do have experience in other professions. I was absolutely shocked at how far behind I have become over the years. Obviously I can operate a computer since I am typing all of this on a laptop. I can perform a lot more functions actually than a lot of people I know. But it seems every job I apply for I need to be proficient in lotus, excel, and spreadsheets. Now I am no dummy by any means but I thought lotus was a type of aquatic plant. I bought some professor software to try to teach me some of this but it is very vague. I know how to do everything else and have tremendous communication and people skills. I have been representing people for many years in a union capacity. As stated earlier I have the Associates in communications and have had prior sales experience. But when it comes to the computer portion of the interview that is where it stops. I pick up on things easily and could be shown but no employer is willing to do this. My communication skills are basically useless and why would I need PEOPLE skills in this day and age. It is more important to be able to devise a pie chart or statistical data evidently so I am vowing to update myself. Many people are in my shoes and the answer is to go back to school. This is an easy answer but not an easy solution. In my job I have forced overtime which means if leave look for a new job. I also need to work some overtime to keep the household running so how can I commit to anything at this point. Unfortunately I am not the only one in this position and most people lose their job and have no idea how to re-enter the work force intelligently. Even though they have many skills they are deemed undesirable. Technology has moved so fast a full time student has a hard time keeping up. If I find myself with this dilemma I am sure there are millions more like me. Workforces need to take the time to update their employees better than they do. They want to move forward but do not want to halt production and give their employees the chance to learn things to better themselves. Some people would not be interested but most would. Employers expect way too much and give way too little. My opinion is what better way to get rid of an employee before retirement age than deem them unable to perform their duties because of the advancement of technology. But they were not offered training or shown how to advance. This is another responsibility of the employee already putting in 60 hours a week just to provide and keep his job. He or she is supposed to find time on their own when there is no time to find. It is a real problem and no one wants to address it or is forced to address it.

I started out my high school career as a buffoon. I decided I didn't want to hit the books and made a joke out of school not trying and playing around. This lasted awhile until I came home with my first report card. I had accumulated 3 D's and an F in algebra. I don't know how this was perceived in most households but in mine it was bad. I remember sitting at the table for dinner and my mom presenting my report card to dad. She usually protected me but she was way mad. She found the most critical time to get me killed and took advantage of it. My dad took one look at it and didn't say a word. He promptly slapped me in the back of the head and said this isn't going to cut it. He proceeded to ground me for one year, took me off the baseball team and made me miserable. I know this is considered abuse now, should have had him put in jail, and sought psychiatric counseling immediately. Back then we knew we had it coming and took our medicine. I know when kids get grounded these days it lasts about 15 minutes, this was not the case. I did not go anywhere but to my room with a book in my hand and a frown on my face. Oddly enough this therapy worked, this ABUSE paid dividends. My grades came up, I still flunked algebra but it was because I was so far behind I couldn't catch up. My sophomore year I proceeded to get an A in algebra and made the honor roll for the most part from there on out. My teachers could not believe the change and wondered what turned it around. It was very simple, a crack in the head, a good old fashioned grounding, and taking away what I lived for, baseball. Time out works for younger kids but as a teenager you have to show them you mean business. I had a version of time out from the ages of 3 to 5 and it was referred to as the bad chair. I hated this chair, it was red and I spent a majority of my time in it. I had to sit in the chair and not leave for being bad. I pushed this issue by keeping my toe touching the chair and reaching for various items I required. My dad allowed this as I think he admired my spunk and creativity. When you are a teenager a little more than the bad chair is required to persuade one from evil activity.

I have to think looking back that hormones play a significant part in our way of thinking as a teenager. It turns us into uncontrollable monsters and we have no idea it is happening. I went to high school in the 80's which was actually a fun time. We dressed comfortably in our parachute pants and basically anything you wore was acceptable no matter how stupid it looked. You could get out of bed and go straight to school because bed head and a little hairspray, was considered cool. The music back then was pretty upbeat with a lot of weird noises in the pop culture. You also had the hair bands that were basically themed toward head banging and rebellion. You had quite a few options to support the mood of the day. Music videos were a hot item and kids would rush home to see Friday Night Videos because no one wanted to miss it. We had a lot of fun then and when we look back it looked like we came from a different planet.

There were so many kids that hated going to school but I actually liked it. I didn't have to go to work and if the grades were up I pretty much did what I wanted. Of course I had to do the chores but that was trivial. I played baseball and loved going to practice so it was a pretty good gig. Why would anyone want to leave it and get shoved into a dog eat dog world? One thing I don't understand is why I was such an ass back in the day. I had a girlfriend that anyone would kill to be with she was such a sweet thing. She loved sports and we had a lot of fun together most of the time, except for when I was being a handful. Her parents were very strict though and we weren't allowed to date for 4 years. Being brain dead from hormones I let this get to me because all my other friends were dating. I loved this girl and it wasn't just puppy love it was the real deal. I was so jealous and immature at times and made it no secret trust me. I would pop somebody in the mouth for even looking at her wrong. I never did anything stupid like get physical with her but I know was intimidating at times. The total opposite of what I am now. Eventually we parted ways I don't blame her, and I don't even get what happened. I am going to blame the hormones because something killed my rational way of thinking. Everyone isn't at fault these days why should I be? My mind went in so many directions at that age, and you don't even realize it. It is a weird time of your life to try to make rhyme or reason of.

I know what you are thinking it wasn't hormones it was the drugs. I can honestly say I never did drugs even though a lot of my friends did. There wasn't any of that peer pressure that you hear about, I just said no I am not doing it. That was good enough for them and didn't really affect me in any way. They didn't FORCE it on me and I didn't really care what they did it was their choice. I was no angel by any means as I would partake in an occasional beverage if available but nothing too serious. I would get in trouble here and there in school because of my lack of rational thinking. I would slap someone around if provoked and I received special counseling for this activity. I think when your hormones are beating each other up inside you have the urge to prove your manhood in some way. I never picked on anyone and got along with classmates but I also made it clear I had limits and not to cross them. The only time I ever backed down was when I got into it with friends. Even though I was brain dead I was smart enough to know if you ever got into a fight with a friend things would never be the same from then on. I would be a chicken in their eyes but I knew it was the best way to keep a friend and I have always cherished my friends to this day.

One of my counseling sessions ended up turning into an in school suspension. This means you sit in the dean's office for the entire day and you couldn't leave. It was a form of punishment as you would even be supervised when going to the bathroom. The activity that produced this sentence was a fishing trip scheduled on school time. My friend Jim coaxed me into thinking that all of our hard work in school constituted a reward. We would suddenly become ill and the therapy would involve a fishing pole and some bait. It was a beautiful day and I remember it well, the blue gill were biting and we were not going to miss out. We headed out in hip waders and were reeling them in left and right. All of the sudden I looked back and saw the driver education car parked up on the bank. I said "uh oh". I saw a pair of waving hands and oddly enough it was the dean of students also enjoying this beautiful day. Maybe he needed a break too! I asked Jim if he saw anything and he said nope. We were stone cold busted at this point and we were going to be punished so why not get what we could out of it. If he wanted us he was going to have to come get us. This would entail wading out about 20 feet to council us on our wrong doing. We decided to chance his desire to apprehend the criminals and finally after about 20 minutes of head shaking and disgust he gave up. We continued to fish and filled our buckets wondering what kind of punishment we were in for. We would have to face it eventually.

As expected the dean was waiting for us the next day and called us in for interrogation. We did what kids do and tried to fib our way out of it. We were experts in this field and even convinced ourselves we were in the right. He unfortunately wasn't buying the huge load of crap spewing from our mouths. Being hormonally brain dead we could not fathom the fact that he thought we were wrong and intended to prosecute. I would later understand why as will be explained. We both received in school suspensions and were to serve our time the next day. What an experience this would be but I would first have to live through what was waiting at home for me now that notification had been given. To my surprise not much was said, after all I was getting good grades and I brought home fish to fry. You have to understand fish in our house was a peacemaker my dad lived to fish and let this one slide.

Jim and I had to sit in the dean's office the entire day and just like prison this leaves idle time for a teenager's mind to think irrationally. The cool part was that everyone that got sent to the office for illicit activity was put on trial with us in the room. There were a lot of cases on tap and we soon understood what this guy went through on a daily basis. This guy was a total screwball and had issues of his own which didn't help matters. Before the afternoon session we had to have lunch as we were allowed a meal, just like prison we had to be fed. Both of us saw this as a time for retribution for the boredom inflicted upon us. We were not allowed to go to the cafeteria because we were in solitary confinement so he had to bring us our lunch. This was a huge mistake in judgment on his part. He brought our lunch trays in and slapped them in front of us. I then announced that I had to have white milk instead of chocolate because it made me sick. This of course was a blatant lie. He gave me a dirty look and went back and got me the white milk I had to have. He slapped the milk down and Jim followed my lead. He wondered where the salt and pepper were. After a huge sigh he went back to the cafeteria and brought him some salt and pepper packets. Each time he slammed the new requirement down a little harder. We knew we had him in Snapsville city limits at this point and I went to the well one more time. I told him we both wanted those little cups of ketchup, how can you eat fries without ketchup? He announced in a very rude tone that this was it! This was the last trip, period! He was not put on this earth to serve us just like my mom would tell me about once a day. We got our ketchup, about thirty of those little cups on a big tray. This was his way of being a smart ass without actually saying it. We took immediate offense to this unprofessional behavior but kept it amongst ourselves until he left. We had all of this left over ketchup it would be a shame to waste it. We knew he would be back to get our trays so we thought it would be fun to line the bottom of the trays thoroughly with it. Sure enough ten minutes later he came back and picked up the trays. Ketchup from the bottom proceeded to run down his arms and coat the cuffs of his very crisp, professional, white shirt. It also managed to penetrate the crevices of his nice gold watch. I have never seen this shade of red in a person's face in my life. Well maybe dad after the garlic incident. He didn't say anything, he couldn't because he always preached just walk away. This was a man now in a very disturbed mood. And this was our last in school suspension. Go figure.

We decided to chill out and let the hornet simmer down in the afternoon. It didn't last long as he left to corral the people that decided to skip last hour. To our luck today he got one! This kid was kind of messed up to begin with, he was a good kid he just had some problems. Actually he hung himself several years ago. The dean got him in the office and the trial began. He asked him where he thought he was going and Tim hesitantly said he had a doctor's appointment. Being fellow teenage liars Jim and I began to giggle and were promptly told to shut up. He asked Tim where the doctor appointment was. After a long moment of silence the response was the hospital. I'm now realizing what this guy goes through in a day weeding though testimony. I have to admit he was no amateur in this regard and played the game well. He asked the name of the doctor and the answer was some oriental guy. He wanted a name and wanted it now. Who could not know the name of the doctor and how could you find him if you didn't know his name? Jim and I are busting at the seams as the heat was really getting put on. Finally Tim blurted out the name Dr. Gookta in desperation. So the dean says let's call the hospital and see if you had an appointment, a crafty move. Tim held his ground and let him call the hospital as he asked for the infamous Dr. Gookta. We all knew it was over at this point but the deal had to be finalized. Of course there was no Dr. Gookta and Tim cracked. He basically begged for mercy of the court at this point which was a huge mistake. He received 3 days of suspension for his crime, harsh punishment I thought. I felt bad because I wondered if the dean didn't have his hands, sleeves, and watch full of ketchup, maybe he would have rendered a lighter sentence.

I graduated High School and worked for a year trying to put a little money back. I then went to the community college full time and worked full time. I wasn't supporting a family and my employer at the furniture store was very flexible on my schedule. I still appreciate that, he was a good man. I wasn't sure what I wanted to do but I knew I loved sports. I decided to pursue radio and television as a career and if anything I would learn to communicate which you need in every job. I hosted the campus television show and did all of the basketball telecast, I absolutely loved it. I did well in my other classes too and graduated with a 3.2 grade point average. Not bad for an algebra flunky. Computers were starting to get hot and I did a lot of work on them but nothing like what is required today. I pursued a career for radio and television for a while and decided I had 2 things going against me. It didn't pay all that well and I had a real problem spontaneously relaying information. This is a talent you have to have and I had issues dealing with it. When it comes to communicating and reading information you won't find anyone better. I have a voice that penetrates, but when it came to being spontaneous on a subject I didn't know about, I locked up. I thought my communication skills in general would be enough to find what I was looking for. I was wrong.

I worked a lot of jobs from this point on bouncing around here and there. I worked some sales jobs that kept me on the road and I decided I didn't want to live like that. My dad was getting increasingly ill so I went to work for the company I am at now for the past 16 years. I decided now that I am in my forties I won't be able to do this physical work when I am 67, the new retirement age, to be 75 by the time I get there. I realize how far behind the times I am and if I had spent the rest of my life paying off college loans I would have that piece of paper stating I am smart. Unfortunately I would still be behind the times and in the same situation, even with a Bachelor's degree. I have so much to offer and have been through life's lessons as you have learned but I don't have the paper saying I am worthy. I blame myself for this but I also blame employers that don't allow their employees the time and training to stay educated as stated earlier. When I originally hired in where I work I had visions of retiring with this company. I enjoyed where I worked and thought it was stable. Then the government and corporate greed took control later on and it is a totally different place. I am doing what most people would do I stay a prisoner at the job I hate so I can provide for my family even though there is no future. Once again the working man or woman gets punished for their loyalty to their company. Sure I have the opportunity to quit and go back to school or take a lesser job, after all this is the land of opportunity I am told. But seriously, who at this point in time would risk losing everything and deprive his or her family to NOT be guaranteed a well-paying job when they graduate? Most if not all people do what I do and remain where they are and hope to retire before they die, which will most likely not happen. For people in this situation it is a dead end street. Employers don't want to educate as a tactic to keep them in captivity. And then they get rid of them because they are uneducated or too old. They never use that excuse they do it another way. They outsource their jobs until they no longer exist or close their doors for a brief time and bring back a cheaper younger workforce. But we should be lucky we have a job with no future and no chance of retirement.

Things are so much different in the school system now than when I went through it. I had a lot of good teachers that went the extra mile with me. I had some that did not care if I keeled over and died in the middle of the room as well. I had a English teacher that clearly took an interest in me and did whatever she could to help me out. I don't think there are too many out there like that anymore from what I have seen. There are a few I have witnessed putting in the time but for the most part they are worried about their state enforced quotas for graduating students. When I got involved with Kathy my future step daughter was around 10 years old. It was pretty evident she wasn't where she needed to be at that stage. Kathy went through a messy divorce and I think some things got neglected of which she will admit. Renee got by and was labeled slow to put it nicely by her educational peers. We worked hard and got her on track by the time she went to High School. I noticed she was continually put in classes that wouldn't challenge her and I became frustrated with this. She was in classes with troubled students and called them dummy classes. She started doing pretty well in school and we wanted to get her into classes that would prepare her for life. The school absolutely refused to do this and we found out later they have a system the school itself gets graded on. If they graduate a percentage they pass, if they failed too many students the school had to answer to it. The school didn't want to risk her failing and it looking bad on their own report card. That is the way to challenge a kid and send a message isn't it? After researching I found out this is a common thing in the school systems. Now we have a kid that is totally unprepared for the job market of today. She is enrolled at the community college and we are hoping for the best for her.

You see on the news every day how we need to educate our kids for the future yet you continue to see cuts hampering it. These teachers hands are tied, not only are they fearful of losing their jobs, they don't receive the funding to do their job correctly. I feel bad for the teachers that have a genuine interest in educating our kids and care about what happens to them. This makes them look bad and they are not to blame. There ARE quality people out there that are being turned away for a cheaper model, and this isn't the place to be corporate. Yet you see Superintendents making six figures who have nothing to do with the everyday relationships between the teachers and the kids. Once again the golden spoon theory is alive and well. Even in our school systems which are one of the most important contributors to our society as well as our future. There are a lot of teachers out there that don't care what happens to these kids too as I explained. These people need to have some accountability and realize how important their jobs are. I have two nieces I am proud to say that are now teachers and I hope they are part of the solution to start turning things around.

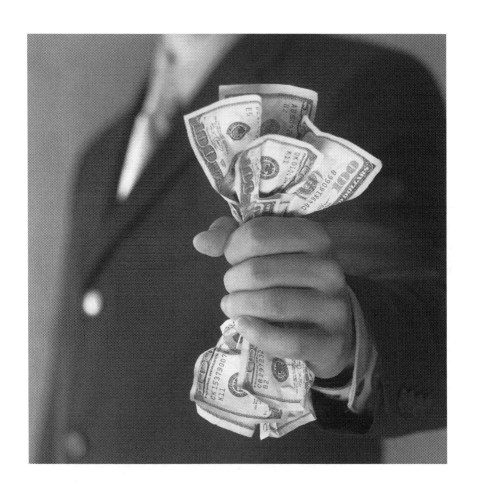

CHAPTER 12

Most people are still proud to be an American in some way. I know from what I see and what I hear that is wearing thin. I hear comments that eventually a rebellion will happen, it will have to. Logically speaking why wouldn't it? It happens all over the world but no one seems to listen. Pompous people don't listen to concerns and don't worry if what they do affects someone down the line. That is what we have running this country, pompous people. We have a president that can get nothing done because of egotistical congressional stalemates. We feed the rest of the world but not our own. We have sick people who can't afford treatment. We have elderly that don't have enough to live on. The list goes on and on. No one wants to talk about it but this country is on the brink of total destruction. Who is going to stop it? Sure if you are rich you can block it out and go about your day but there is going to be a point where greed comes to a halt. It may be long after I am gone but it appears to a lot of people it isn't too far off.

There are so many references to 2012 here in the past year or so. I think the only one who determines our destiny is god himself. I do believe though eventually the earth will find a way to cleanse itself of the damage we have created. I also feel we are getting to that point soon. We have created huge oil spills, massive pollution, wild fires, greenhouse emissions, and we keep adding to the list. I believe we are getting signs that we had better change our ways and quickly. Tsunami's, earthquakes, and hurricanes, arctic glaciers, something is telling us to get our act together. What I don't understand is how someone even if they aren't concerned for themselves, what about their kids and grandkids? A little more is getting done to appease the tree huggers and get some votes but it isn't enough and there is no sense of urgency. Everything will break down eventually if you push it to the limit long enough and that is what we are doing. Not just this country, every country. I guess all we can do is wait it out and watch everyone say "what do we do now" after it happens. Just like New Orleans only a million times worse.

I realize life is not always a Leave it to Beaver episode and no matter what there will be a rotten part on the apple. There will always be greed, corruption, crime, pollution, and people that just don't care. This has happened throughout history and it always will. I don't understand though when it gets to a certain point the world doesn't work diligently to get it under control. Get a handle on these things before they happen instead of after. Enforce strict regulations and spend money on waste control and what to do about it. Prioritize what is important and realize padding pockets is at the bottom of the list. Create some positives for the people of your country and perhaps you will see an attitude change and more participation. Everyone is important even at the bottom treat them that way.

There is a serious misconception out there that people who live on less also think less. I have learned valuable lessons in life that everyone has something to contribute in some way. Some of the smartest people I know can't operate a computer, not because they couldn't, they haven't been taught. I entered my apprenticeship thinking I was one smart cookie when I found out I was one misinformed cookie. I worked with a hillbilly for some of my training, he had that twang in his voice, used the word aint in every sentence. I have worked with corporate people being a district manager and these were some intelligent people let me tell you. They took no shame in telling you they knew it all and frowned on people in a working capacity. I heard the comments of cave men and retards all the time it infuriated me. I want to inform you that this moonshine drinking hillbilly was one of the smartest people I have ever met. He could put these over educated, egotistical, self-centered, arrogant, jerks in the ground. This guy could calculate anything, geometry, calculus, trigonometry, you name it. He could run pipe for a mile with twist and turns and it would come out perfect on a dime. He could weld anything and make it look unbelievable I was astounded by this guy. These supposed geniuses wouldn't even know where to begin and they refer to working men as retards. He would fix countless engineering blunders and make it right but this guy was the cave man. What a lesson for a young punk like me to learn even though I already knew it. Our society is based on perception and not fact. Everyone has something to offer it just might be different from what society deems as important. It is a common saying with engineering that it looks good on paper but it never works in the real world. This is true a majority of the time but never admitted to. A book can teach you but it can't show you and the same goes in the way the world works. We have too many people putting it on paper and not enough making it work.

This country has a way of labeling people important or unimportant. I look at it as everyone is important and you can learn from each individual. Would you want the President of Ford working on your car or a mechanic? Which would you consider more important if your car broke down? One makes millions and one barely gets by if they are lucky. Would you want one of the executive board members of a power company working on your power lines after an ice storm or the guy who works on them every day? One has a million dollar home and the other has a small home he will most likely never pay for. There was a time that the people who keep the nation running were respected and actually compensated for their importance. Evidently those people aren't important anymore.

We have such a variety of personalities here in the U.S. and the majority being upstanding citizens but we also have that rotten part of the apple. What makes one part more rotten than the other? One part robs a liquor store one part robs your pension and social security but they are viewed as distinctly different. One rots in a jail cell for stealing a couple hundred bucks and the other buys a private jet for stealing millions. A thief is a thief any way you cut it and it is about time it is treated as such. This is a good place to start the cleansing process. We have always been taught to start at the bottom and work your way to the top. It is now time to reverse that thinking and start at the top where the problem lies and work your way to the bottom.

I thought about taking the egghead approach to this book and quote a bunch of statistics but I have a problem with that. I hear a different statistic for everything known to man. It all depends on who you want to listen to. Every poll is different from one party to the next and no one knows who to believe. The people I am relating to here don't need numbers to convince them. They live it every day. They see it all around, they see it in their paychecks, in their mailbox full of bills, the prices at the gas pump and the grocery store. We are beyond having to put a number behind what is going on and are tired of hearing about it. We are not that stupid! We all know the wealth in this country goes to a small group and we get the scraps.

PERIOD! The scraps are expected to pay the taxes, feed the hungry, cure the sick, pay for the technology. Enough is enough it is time to bleed the top for a change and not the bottom.

Controlling bonuses for anyone making 200k would be a good start. If someone makes this kind of money on a yearly basis is a bonus necessary? If you work 5 years you have made a million dollars, wow tough to make it on that. This money would be put back into wages, a defined pension, and healthcare where it should be to begin with. There is no reason for a defined pension to be abolished. I know they are expensive I have worked with them. When you see this amount of money dealt out on a yearly basis at the top there is no excuse to not keep them funded. It is purely greed. There needs to be a salary cap on CEO's and their hand-picked executive boards. There is no way a worker should be without the basic necessities of life while another uses hundred dollar bills for wiping their ass. I am not opposed to a bonus completely, if the employees get them and the upper crust has criteria to receive theirs. How about a bonus not being based on what the employees accomplish but what is accomplished FOR the employees. If a company keeps a pension funded, reasonable health insurance, paid time off, a middle income based salary they then would receive a REASONABLE BONUS. This is in reference to ALL workers top to bottom. If they keep the jobs on our soil they would be rewarded as well. It makes me sick even saying this because it is something they should be doing already without incentives. If a company is in financial trouble the salaries at the very top get cut first by a significant amount before any layoff of employees can take place. This would be the only way to make someone think twice about eliminating jobs to pad their own pocket. Companies need to be held accountable and if they want to send the jobs overseas make them pay dearly for it. The word TAX is a very powerful word and it is about time we started using it for people other than the poor chaps working like a dog for peanuts. I know you have to regulate all of this and that is pretty tough when the regulators are a big part of the problem. I'm not Republican, I'm not democrat anymore either. I am pissed off. I don't care if the president is black, white, yellow, man, woman, republican, democrat, somebody has got to get control and fast. The masses are getting angrier by the minute and there is trouble on the horizon.

I understand the cost of health care is absolutely ignorant and the cost of workers compensation insurance is out the roof. I am sympathetic with amount of money the employer has to pay for these necessities. This never should have gotten to the point that it has and we can thank the evil lawyers for that. Every time I fart or blow my nose there is a new lawsuit going forward. Workers get lawyers from my experiences because the employer's compensation insurance refuse to pay the medical bills for individuals injured at work. If the bills were paid there wouldn't be an issue and that would be that. The bills don't get paid so the worker has no choice but to get a lawyer and the insurance company ends up paying the bills, the injured, and the lawyer. They in turn get back by jacking the insurance rates up on the company. The insurance gets their money back and more. The company then gets it back in the form of wages, retirement, etc. The bottom of the food chain again gets the short end. I realize there are people who work so they don't have to work. In other words they try to play the system and make money off of the companies insurance in the form of a settlement claim. I can tell you though there is an extremely low percentage and even fewer that get away with it. I kind of see it as one thief, the insurance, stealing from another thief, the companies, in a nutshell. There is one more part of the equation and that is us with a nice new pay cut and an old empty wallet.

Have you ever been in the hospital and taken a look at the itemized bill? I hope you never have to deal with it but take a peek at one sometime. You will be amazed at the art of fleecing that takes place while you are sick. Take a look at how much a pair of those 10 cent rubber gloves or a can of 7 up will cost you. Most likely you will notice that many doctors you never see or speak to are getting paid off of your chart. I hate going to the doctor because I can never get away with just one visit. It is always see this doctor, that doctor, pay for a bunch of test you don't need. Then they want you back in two days, a week, then two weeks, then a month. It is amazing how much the flu can cost you. I understand they can't just wave a magic wand and figure out the ailment but the patient should be able to decide how much they want to put into it. After the bills are run up to staggering amounts the insurance company fights it first to try to get you to pay more, pays their part if you are lucky, and promptly raises the rates to get the money back with interest. It is a never ending cycle and everyone gets their return except the person who had the flu. I know that is just the way it is these days. We aren't smart enough to figure it out so just pay it and shut up. The great part is the people we need to fight this get their healthcare taken care of. Why would they worry about someone who has no insurance or not enough money to pay the premiums and co-pay's. I am not even going into medicare, I could argue about that for days. Why pay for the elderly, if they die that is just less that has to be paid in the long run right? That helps defer the cost in egghead terms. You know this is part of the thinking process as disgusting as it is. It is all about statistics and the bottom line. Insurance should be defined as screwing you with a smile on their face. If they weren't making money they wouldn't be in business would they? The less they pay the more they play whether you are in pain or not. They care about you because the commercials say so, just be happy with that. Our government obviously is content with it.

The government is also content with borrowing on our so called entitlements like social security. It is amazing the word entitlement is used on something that we spend our entire working lives paying for. It is good to know I am entitled to something that goes out of my check every week for my retirement. The better part is we aren't even going to get it because the government felt the need to tap into it. It is so nice to know that the greatest country in the world can take the liberty anytime they want to steal from the people who make it great. I know that stealing is a very uneducated term to use but it is better than the obscene term I would like to use in this case. I am sure the government would use a financial term way over our heads to describe stealing but I think we are a little smarter than they give us credit for. We can all rest easy knowing that the money is going for a good cause, bail outs for the rich, free health care for government officials, outrageous retirement packages, you know all the necessities. Like I said there is no need to go into statistics, I unlike your government know you are smart enough to realize it. I know I am so sick of all the red tape and insignificant numbers I could throw up as we speak. The time has passed for analyzing the time has come for fixing it. I have a pile of numbers sitting next to me but what is the point. It is time to quit speaking in terms of numbers and in terms of people. We know millions are out of work, millions can't pay the bills, millions can't afford health care, and millions won't retire. There are your statistics what more is needed? The government gets paid to do a job, now quit the bickering and DO IT!

I have spent most of my working years trying to fight for worker's rights. There are so many people like myself that have been shunned by other working people after years of public brainwashing. I speak for myself here but I know they would agree. Just because I have the word Union in my title does not mean I don't think about the person at the Supercenter getting paid half of what they should. I think of everyone out there that goes to work every day. This isn't about company or union it is about people. People who bash unions at a lower level want to bring them DOWN to their wage and want them to NOT get what they are NOT getting. This is not the goal here. The goal is to bring every working person UP to where they should be. The company you work for is making millions why shouldn't the workers be able to make a living? Unions were made to band people together to ensure the dream for us and our children. It doesn't matter if you are washing cars, a receptionist, lab worker, data-entry you are a part of the workforce in this country. You should be treated with respect and be compensated for what you do. This is the message that we are trying to convey. Our government can't get together and solve anything obviously so guess who will have to do it? The people, specifically the working people of a lower class are the ones that will ultimately have to get it done. Whether you are union or non-union it doesn't matter. We all need to support each other and find out a way to get back what is rightfully ours. You have seen countries fighting back against their government and the rich with violence in the news every day recently. The only way of fighting back the right way is the ballot box. But what happens when this doesn't work? Most people do not feel good about the candidates they simply vote for the lesser of the two evils. I remember when people would get into heated arguments about being republican or democrat. Now I hear it doesn't matter they are all crooks no matter who you vote for. There is beginning to be less and less separation between the two parties in people's eyes. Sure you still have people that will vote by party but it is diminishing. People are sick of promises that are not kept and seeing our country go down the toilet. What happens when it gets to a point of no return?

I am hoping that if people read and heed this book we can avoid the inevitable, anarchy. People on a higher level laugh about it and shrug it off, it will never happen. My question is just how long can society be pushed when MOST working people lose everything they have? Individuals become unstable and bad things happen. Hatred and desperation are strong human emotions and you see it brought out when people lose their jobs, homes, and ability to provide. What will happen when a majority is put in this situation? You will see more crime than can be controlled. Violence is never a way to solve anything and it should never get to that but no one seems to be concerned. At least the boys at the top aren't worried. History supports that when minorities of unhappy people become a majority it creates destruction. We have to stop being blind to what is out there and take control. We need to do whatever it takes to avoid an internal war among the people and continue to band together a little more at a time. We have to take it upon ourselves to be the voice of reason and provide for one another. A job our government should be doing. If someone is in a fight to get or keep what is rightfully theirs join the fight. We are the only ones that can keep the sanity and change things the right way. If not the war won't be in Afghanistan or Iraq, it will be here. I hear it all the time and people are thinking it. Let's get it together before the thinking turns into doing. In the past we have seen riots by a limited number of people. What happens when those numbers start growing because more people have nothing and join in? It is instinct to do what you have to in order to survive and once rational people could turn to this. I hope to God above this never happens but it is becoming reality as each year goes by. It will only take one event to set it off in one part of the country and it will happen in another. We have seen it before in small quantities but not what it could evolve into. We need to eliminate even the possibility of it starting. There are so many people involved in our food processing it only takes one angry individual to affect the lives of so many people. The Tylenol tampering sent the country in a panic because of one angry person. That person may still be out there plotting another strike no one knows. We spend countless hours criticizing other countries as we watch them rebel after being pushed too far. In this country people tend to act a little more discreetly and in a more calculated fashion. We are so worried about terrorism we are headed down the same road and not even thinking about our own people getting even. Companies and the government keep taking and eventually someone is going to be pushed to the limit and take things to the next level. That would never happen here, would it? It happens on a smaller scale every day and that is bad enough. People who decide to get even here affect people that generally have nothing to do with it because they are the easiest to access. The poor sap that just happens to be at the mall that day takes the bullet over what someone else did to the shooter. This never makes any sense to me. How does killing an innocent person solve anything? It sends a message but what message? You can screw me but I am going to take it out on someone else? Violence is a no win situation but people think it is the only way you can get things done or get even.

Technology is going to lead to the death of many people I am afraid. The internet is giving the knowledge and ability to people that shouldn't have it. It opens a line of communication to people you normally wouldn't know existed. You can learn things you should not know how to do, get things you shouldn't be able to, it is creating the ability to form alliances. The bad part is it does so many good things so people want it. You can find that mower part you can't find anywhere else. You can talk to the people you haven't spoken to in years. You can find a job you never knew was available. The good things you can do outweigh the bad so you will never see it go away. It will only go more widespread. You cannot control what happens on it although the government tries. The internet gives free reign for people to do whatever they want whenever they want. This is not a bad thing for the normal everyday person like me or you. Unfortunately no one can decide who is normal and who is not. People can find out how to build a bomb, contaminate food and water, it will show you how to kill people without detection. Basically the internet is a handbook on how to destroy the world as we know it. And anyone can get it. This is pretty scary stuff in my opinion.

I referred to molestation earlier and you always see the predator shows where they catch somebody in the act. How many don't get caught and use it as a tool to find what they need? How many people get their lives taken financially from some internet scheme? How many people get their identities stolen like I did? To me there are more cons than pros but what are you going to do? Internet is now a part of our life we cannot do without so it will never leave. It is one of those hidden dangers like asbestos that is killing us and we don't even know it. The internet is supposed to make life easier but the world was a much better place when it didn't exist. It was less convenient but I think I would gladly go back to the way it was.

We also cannot live without the use of a cell phone. I have one of course and now 5 year olds have them. They are a great thing but they also have you by the kahunas if you think about it. You get locked into these contracts and if something happens you can no longer pay for it, too bad pay up. As a parent you want your kids to have it for safety reasons. If something goes wrong they can call someone no matter where they are at and this is good. They can also have their head buried in it 24/7 instead of doing schoolwork or sleeping this is bad. I can't count the number of parents that have been furious with a 600 dollar unexpected phone bill. You want them to have it in case something happens but you can't trust them to be responsible with it. This is quite a dilemma and you bet someone is out there taking advantage of it. You pay for an unlimited everything package to counter the fleecing of your wallet but if you add it up you are paying just as much. If you get angry and want to shut it off it will cost you a ridiculous amount. The parent can't win they are a hostage of technology whether they can afford it or not. Parents always fear their child will be abducted or be stranded somewhere. They know the first question that will be asked if something bad happens is does the child have a cell phone. How is the perception of the parent viewed if they don't? Again they are cheap and don't care about their kid. I will say I like the fact that you can find someone through the phone and help solve crimes by placing people here or there at certain times. But as a person who doesn't engage in criminal activity it kind of makes me feel like I have a chip in my head at all times. I feel weird about that, maybe it is just me. I don't like the feeling of being tracked like a tagged anaconda in the rain forest. You can bet someone is using this technology to do bad things and it makes it so much easier to carry out a plan of destruction. The inconvenient pay phone is no longer in the equation like you see in the movies. The cell phone is also another part of our culture that will never leave with our dependence on it. The thought of taking them would create a riot in itself. Being advanced can create power but it also creates weakness because no one knows how to live life without things like the internet and the cell phone. Who has the power? It isn't us.

The media is also a downfall that has really influenced how society works. I absolutely love television, I have studied it and I watch a lot of it. Television has been a staple of the American family for many years but just like everything else it has changed. It used to be a device to send a message of morality and decency. It is now used to see who can do something worse than the other. For example it is used to portray how one country is in absolute shambles and how great we have things here. It convinces people to wave that flag proudly just what the government wants. When you see how bad things are somewhere else you tend to think the bad things they are doing to you here are nothing. It is the same as that you are lucky to have a job theory. We only see the pictures of the sick and the hungry but don't we have sick and hungry here? I would be a fool to say we don't have it better than some countries because we do but I don't need to be manipulated to believe it. There are countries with happy people, less crime rates, cleaner environments, but you rarely see that portrayed only the negative. We have become pompous in that way of thinking because the average person only knows what is viewed on television. I always hear how Arabic television never tells the whole story when we are at war with them. I would be shocked if we weren't looked at in the same eyes. Every country believes what they see and hear in their own media outlet, now that is power! There is a high level of trust there and it should be that way but with the money being thrown around these days I have become leery of anything. I am not saying we are lied to I am saying we don't see and hear everything to make sure that "banner yet wave". The media builds a degree of hatred that cultivates a patriotic bond among its citizens. The government uses it to their advantage as much as possible, you hear it every speech on every newscast. This takes the heat off them and puts it somewhere else. That is when the dirty work begins while your focus is off of them and on the bad guy.

What a bleak view from the eyes of the common person isn't it? I have spent most of my life listening and filing comments and information in my own computer, my mind. I wrote this book for two reasons, to relate to people, and voice opinions that aren't getting out there. I know that "regular" people are frustrated that their point of view sits in the pits of their stomachs and never gets relayed. We live in a free country unless it offends someone then we can't say it. We can have things crammed down our throats like using the word Holiday instead of Christmas, foreigners taking our jobs, burning the American flag, trying to abolish the pledge of allegiance. We have to be compassionate to what others think and believe but it doesn't work both ways. There are many law abiding citizens of different origins and sexuality that do care and do the right things. They contribute to their best and don't expect for us change our lives for their customs and beliefs. Most of them fit right in and become a part of us and we appreciate them for who they are. There are others that are not happy until we change to suit their specific lifestyle and this is where many people have an issue.

Government is supposed to work for all people not just wealthy people and this has got to change. This country is like a winding clock and all the parts have to be cohesive to work. Each part has a specific function and no part is more important than the other. This country has not worked cohesively for quite some time and we are all starting to see the affects. We need to get this clock wound back up and all the parts working so we can have a future for all that live here. This doesn't mean we all have to be rich, it means we all have to be given the tools to make our part work. Those tools are security, family time, and a retirement to enjoy things. If you throw in taking care of our own sick, hungry, and elderly you have got a start. Share the wealth and things will change.

I shared my ups and downs, some opinions and some childhood stories in hoping you might get to know me along the way. I wanted you to get some insight of how I think about the simple things and the complex as well. I also have attempted to be the voice for those who don't have a voice. The basic theme is that we are all concerned about what happens in the future years and we are the only people that can change it. We are at the point we can't point fingers anymore and have to take action. There is no time to waste. God bless you all.